The
Complete Guide
to
ATKINS DIET
2024

A Step by Step Guide for a Low-Carb Lifestyle || Over 100 Easy and Delicious Low-Carb Recipes for a Healthier You

Dr. Jim Davis

Copyright © 2024 Dr. Jim Davis

CONTENTS

Chapter Five: 28 Day Meal Plan

INTRODUCTION

Marie was always self-conscious about her weight. She had tried many different diets over the years, but nothing seemed to work for her. She felt like she was stuck in a cycle of losing weight and gaining it back. One day, she stumbled upon a cookbook for the Atkins Diet online. The book promised easy, delicious, low-carb recipes that would help her lose weight and keep it off. Marie decided to give it a try. She was surprised by how much she enjoyed the recipes, and how easy they were to follow.

Within a few weeks, Marie began to see results. She felt more energetic, her clothes were starting to fit more loosely, and she was feeling more confident. The cookbook not only provided healthy recipes, but also tips for maintaining a low-carb lifestyle. Marie realized that she could still enjoy her favorite foods, just in a healthier way. As she continued to follow the Atkins Diet, she found that her cravings for unhealthy foods began to diminish. She was able to control her appetite and make better choices about what she ate.

In just a few months, Marie had lost over 15 pounds and felt like a new person. She was surprised at how much her energy level had increased and how much better she felt overall. The Atkins Diet had not only helped her to lose weight, but it had also changed her relationship with food. She no longer felt controlled by her cravings and felt like she was finally in control of her health. The cookbook had not only provided healthy recipes, but it had also given her the tools to make lasting lifestyle changes.

This book is designed to provide you with everything you need to know about the Atkins Diet, including how it works, the benefits it offers, and how to follow it. The Atkins Diet is not just another fad diet - it's a proven method for losing weight and improving your health. In fact, over 40 years of research has shown that it's effective for weight loss, improving blood sugar control, and reducing the risk of heart disease.

With this book, you'll learn how to make healthy food choices that will help you reach your weight loss goals. You'll discover which foods to enjoy, which to limit, and which to avoid altogether. And with the meal plans, shopping lists, and recipes in this book, you'll have everything you need to make the Atkins Diet work for you. If you're ready to make a change and get serious about your health, the Atkins Diet is the way to go. And this book is the perfect companion for your journey. So what are you waiting for? Start reading and start losing weight today!

LOW-CARBS

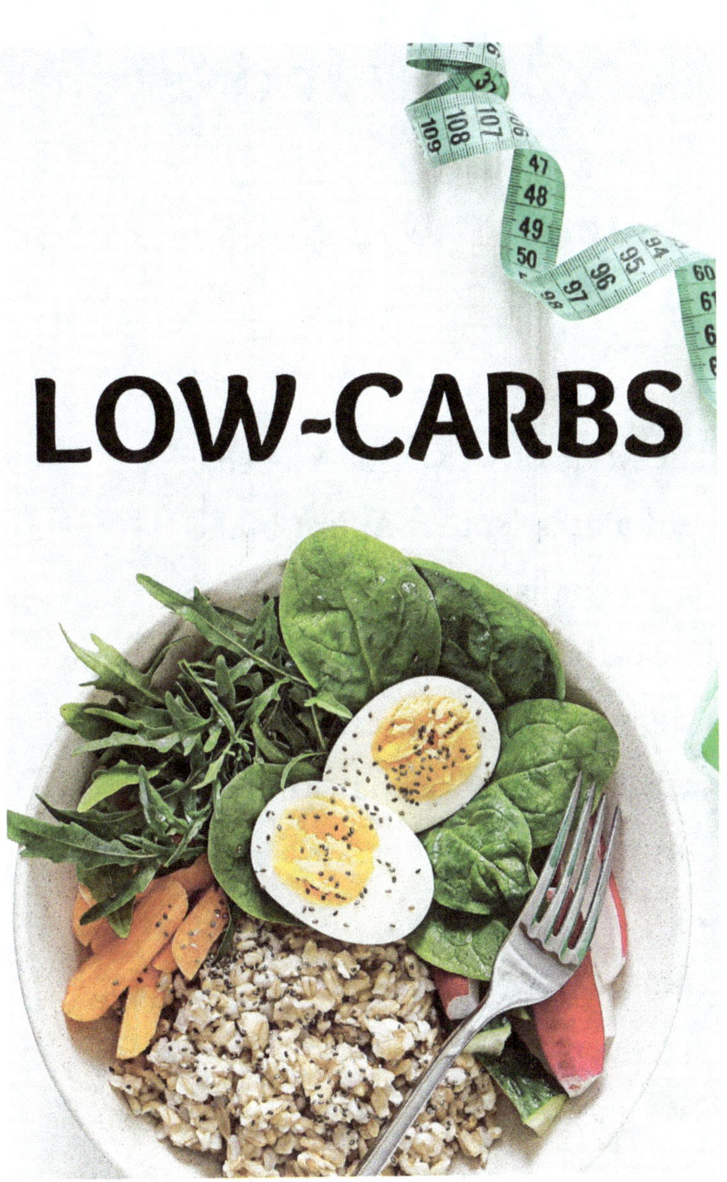

CHAPTER ONE

Understanding the Science of Atkins Diet

The Atkins Diet was developed by cardiologist Robert Atkins in the 1970s. He observed that patients who followed a low-carbohydrate diet had success losing weight. His theory was that by restricting carbohydrates, the body would switch from burning glucose (sugar) for energy to burning fat, a process known as ketosis. This led to weight loss, improved blood sugar control, and other health benefits. Over the years, the Atkins Diet has been updated and refined, and is now widely recognized as an effective tool for weight loss and health.

The Atkins Diet is based on the science of ketosis. Ketosis is a metabolic state in which your body burns fat for fuel, instead of carbohydrates. On the Atkins Diet, you eat a low-carbohydrate, high-fat diet. This causes your body to switch from burning carbs for fuel to burning fat. As your body switches to burning fat, it begins to produce molecules called ketones. Ketones are produced in the liver from fat and are used as an energy source. This process of burning fat and producing ketones is called ketosis.

How the Atkins Diet Works

The Atkins diet is a low-carbohydrate eating plan designed to promote weight loss and improve overall health. The Atkins Diet works by controlling your insulin levels. Insulin is a hormone that helps to regulate blood sugar levels. When you eat carbohydrates, your body breaks them down into glucose, which raises your blood sugar levels. Your body then produces insulin to lower your blood sugar levels. However, if you eat too many carbs, your body will produce too much insulin, which can cause weight gain. By restricting carbs on the Atkins Diet, you'll keep your insulin levels low, which can help you lose weight.

The Atkins Diet is sometimes referred to as a low-carbohydrate, high-fat (LCHF) diet. While many people think of fat as the enemy, the Atkins Diet recognizes that certain types of fat can be beneficial for your health. The diet focuses on eating healthy fats, such as monounsaturated and polyunsaturated fats, which can help reduce inflammation and improve heart health. Foods that are high in healthy fats include avocados, olive oil, nuts, and seeds. The Atkins Diet also discourages eating unhealthy fats, such as trans fats and saturated fats, which can increase your risk of heart disease.

In general, the Atkins Diet works by using a combination of carbohydrate restriction and calorie control to promote weight loss. Carbohydrate restriction helps to keep your insulin levels low, which in turn helps to control your appetite and prevent cravings. Calorie control helps to ensure that you're not eating too many calories, which can lead to weight gain. The Atkins Diet also focuses on eating whole, unprocessed foods, which can help you feel more satisfied and avoid overeating. Finally, the Atkins Diet also encourages regular exercise, which is an important part of any healthy lifestyle.

Benefits of a Low-Carb Lifestyle

A low-carb lifestyle, like the Atkins Diet, can offer a variety of health benefits. Some of the main benefits include;

Weight Loss

One of the primary benefits is weight loss. Low-carb diets like the Atkins Diet have been shown to be effective for weight loss, even when compared to low-fat diets. By reducing carbohydrate intake, the body shifts to burning stored fat for energy, leading to a more efficient fat-burning process.

Improved Blood Sugar Control

Low-carb diets can help stabilize blood sugar levels, making them beneficial for people with diabetes or insulin resistance. By minimizing spikes in blood sugar, it can also reduce the risk of developing type 2 diabetes.

Increased Energy Levels

When you eat a high-carb diet, your body relies on glucose for energy. This can cause blood sugar levels to spike and crash, leading to energy crashes. A low-carb diet can help to stabilize blood sugar levels, leading to more consistent energy levels throughout the day. Many people report feeling more energetic and alert on a low-carb diet, as they experience fewer blood sugar crashes and more consistent energy throughout the day.

Reduced Cravings

Cutting back on carbohydrates can help reduce cravings for sugary and starchy foods. This can make it easier to stick to a healthy eating plan and avoid overeating.

Better Mental Clarity

Research has shown that low-carb diets can increase levels of BDNF, a protein that plays a role in brain function. BDNF is involved in processes like memory, learning, and mood. A low-carb diet can help to balance neurotransmitters like serotonin, which can improve mood and reduce feelings of depression and anxiety. This combination of improved brain function and mood can lead to greater mental clarity and focus.

Improved Heart Health

Low-carb diets can lead to improvements in various markers of heart health, such as lower triglyceride levels, increased HDL (good) cholesterol, and reduced blood pressure.

Better Digestive Health

Cutting out processed carbs and sugar can improve digestive health by reducing inflammation and promoting a healthier balance of gut bacteria. Some people also report that the Atkins Diet can help to improve symptoms of digestive disorders like irritable bowel syndrome (IBS). This may be due to the fact that a low-carb diet can help to reduce bloating and gas, two common symptoms of IBS.

Management of Certain Health Conditions

Low-carb diets have been associated with positive outcomes in conditions such as polycystic ovary syndrome (PCOS), metabolic syndrome, and epilepsy. Always consult with a healthcare professional before making significant dietary changes, especially if you have pre-existing health conditions.

CHAPTER TWO

Phases of the Atkins Diet

The Atkins Diet offers a structured approach to weight loss and maintenance through its distinct phases. By gradually transitioning the body into a state of ketosis and controlling carbohydrate intake, individuals can achieve sustainable weight loss and improve their overall health over time.

Central to the Atkins Diet are its distinct phases, each designed to gradually transition individuals into a state of ketosis, where the body burns fat for fuel. Understanding these phases is crucial for

effectively implementing the Atkins Diet
and achieving desired results.

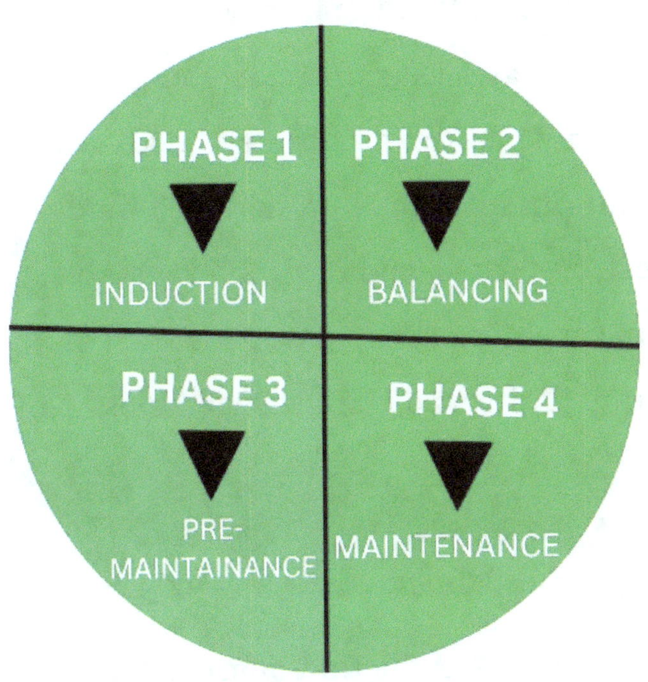

Induction Phase

The first phase of the Atkins Diet is known
as the Induction phase. Lasting around two

weeks, its primary goal is to kickstart weight loss by severely restricting carbohydrate intake to 20-25 grams per day. During this phase, the body shifts from using carbohydrates as its primary energy source to burning stored fat for fuel. Foods allowed in this phase include protein-rich foods like meat, fish, eggs, and low-carb vegetables while avoiding high-carb foods such as grains, fruits, and starchy vegetables.

Balancing Phase

Following the Induction phase is the Balancing phase, where carbohydrate intake is gradually increased to a level where weight loss continues steadily. This phase typically lasts until individuals are within 10 pounds of their target weight. Carbohydrate intake is slowly increased in 5-gram increments each week, primarily from nutrient-dense sources like fruits, nuts, and whole grains. The focus remains on controlling carbohydrate intake while continuing to lose weight at a sustainable pace.

Pre-Maintenance Phase

Once individuals are nearing their goal weight, they transition to the Pre-Maintenance phase. In this phase, carbohydrate intake is further increased to determine the maximum amount that can be consumed without gaining weight. This phase helps individuals identify their carbohydrate tolerance level, which varies depending on factors such as metabolism, activity level, and individual physiology. It encourages long-term adherence to a balanced diet while still enjoying a wider variety of foods.

Maintenance Phase

The Maintenance phase is the final stage of the Atkins Diet and focuses on sustaining weight loss and overall health in the long term. By this point, individuals have reached their target weight and have established a stable eating pattern that works for them. Carbohydrate intake is adjusted based on individual needs and lifestyle factors, with an emphasis on whole, nutrient-rich foods to support overall well-being. Regular monitoring and adjustments may be necessary to maintain weight loss and prevent regaining excess pounds.

CHAPTER THREE

Choose the Right Foods

Choosing the right foods while following the Atkins diet is crucial for achieving optimal results. It involves a balance of proteins, fats, and carbohydrates while adhering to the principles of the different phases. Prioritizing nutrient-dense, whole foods and staying hydrated are essential components for success. By understanding which foods to prioritize and which to limit, individuals can effectively manage their weight and improve their overall health on the Atkins diet.

1. Focus on Protein

Protein is a cornerstone of the Atkins diet as it helps maintain muscle mass and promotes satiety. Opt for high-quality sources of protein such as poultry, fish, eggs, tofu, and lean cuts of beef or pork. Incorporating protein into each meal can help keep you feeling full and satisfied while stabilizing blood sugar levels.

2. Healthy Fats

Unlike traditional low-fat diets, the Atkins diet encourages the consumption of healthy fats to provide energy and support various bodily functions. Include sources of healthy fats such as avocados, nuts, seeds, olive oil, and fatty fish like salmon and sardines.

These fats not only add flavor to meals but also help keep you feeling full and satisfied.

3. Non-Starchy Vegetables

Non-starchy vegetables are low in carbohydrates and high in fiber, making them an excellent choice for the Atkins diet. Aim to fill your plate with colorful vegetables such as leafy greens, broccoli, cauliflower, peppers, zucchini, and Brussels sprouts. These vegetables provide essential vitamins, minerals, and antioxidants without significantly impacting blood sugar levels.

4. Limit Carbohydrates

While following the Atkins diet, it's essential to limit the intake of high-carbohydrate foods such as grains, starchy vegetables, fruits, and sugary treats. Instead, focus on low-carb options such as leafy greens, cruciferous vegetables, berries, and other low-sugar fruits in moderation. By reducing carbohydrate intake, the body shifts into a state of ketosis, where it burns fat for fuel, leading to weight loss.

5. Monitor Portion Sizes

Even though certain foods are allowed on the Atkins diet, it's essential to monitor portion sizes to control calorie intake and ensure balanced nutrition. Pay attention to serving sizes and listen to your body's hunger cues to prevent overeating.

6. Stay Hydrated

Adequate hydration is essential for overall health and can also support weight loss on the Atkins diet. Drink plenty of water throughout the day and consider incorporating herbal teas or flavored sparkling water for variety.

Foods To Avoid

To adhere to the principles of the Atkins Diet, it's essential to avoid certain foods high in carbohydrates. Here are some foods to avoid:

1. *Sugary Foods:* Eliminate or significantly reduce the intake of sugary foods and beverages, including

candies, pastries, cakes, cookies, and sugary drinks. These can cause spikes in blood sugar levels.

2. *Grains and Cereals:* Avoid grains and cereals such as wheat, rice, oats, and barley. This includes products made from these grains like bread, pasta, and breakfast cereals, as they are high in carbohydrates.

3. *Starchy Vegetables:* Limit starchy vegetables like potatoes, corn, and peas, as they contain higher amounts of carbohydrates. Opt for non-starchy vegetables instead.

4. *Fruits High in Sugar:* While fruits are generally healthy, some are high in natural sugars. Avoid or limit fruits like bananas, grapes, and mangoes.

Choose berries or other low-carb fruits in moderation.

5. *Legumes and Beans:* Beans, lentils, and other legumes are rich in carbohydrates. They should be restricted on the Atkins Diet due to their carb content.

6. *Processed and Packaged Foods:* Many processed and packaged foods contain hidden sugars and carbohydrates. Avoid items like pre-packaged snacks, sauces, and dressings that may have added sugars.

7. *High-Carb Dairy:* Be cautious with dairy products as some can be higher in carbohydrates. Limit milk and choose full-fat, low-carb options like cheese and cream.

8. ***Alcohol and Sweetened Beverages:***
    Alcoholic beverages and sweetened
    drinks should be limited or avoided as
    they often contain sugars and can
    interfere with ketosis.

9. ***Certain Nuts and Seeds:*** While nuts
    and seeds are generally allowed on the
    Atkins Diet, some are higher in carbs.
    Limit cashews and pistachios, and opt
    for lower-carb options like almonds
    and walnuts.

10. ***Low-Fat or Diet Products:*** Avoid
    low-fat or diet products, as they often
    replace fats with sugars to enhance
    flavor. Stick to natural fats for satiety.

CHAPTER FOUR

Meal Planning and Recipes

Meal planning in the Atkins diet involves carefully selecting foods that are low in carbohydrates while emphasizing protein and healthy fats. Preparing low-carb meals and snacks can help you succeed on the Atkins diet while enjoying a variety of delicious and satisfying foods. Here's how you can plan meals within the framework of the Atkins diet:

1. *Focus on Protein:* As discussed in the previous chapter, include a source of protein in every meal. This could be poultry, fish,

eggs, tofu, or lean meats like beef or pork. Protein helps keep you feeling full and satisfied, which can aid in weight loss.

2. ***Choose Low-Carb Vegetables:*** Incorporate non-starchy vegetables like leafy greens, broccoli, cauliflower, zucchini, and peppers. These vegetables are high in fiber and nutrients but low in carbohydrates, making them suitable for the Atkins diet.

3. ***Include Healthy Fats:*** Add sources of healthy fats such as avocado, olive oil, nuts, and seeds to your meals. These fats provide essential nutrients and help keep you satiated.

4. *Limit Carbohydrates:* Be mindful of carbohydrate intake and opt for low-carb alternatives. Avoid high-carb foods like bread, pasta, rice, and sugary snacks. Instead, choose low-carb options like cauliflower rice, spiralized vegetables, or lettuce wraps.

5. *Plan Balanced Meals:* Aim for a balance of protein, healthy fats, and low-carb vegetables in each meal. This balance helps stabilize blood sugar levels and promotes satiety.

6. *Stay Hydrated:* Drink plenty of water throughout the day to stay hydrated and support overall health.

7. *Snack Wisely:* Choose low-carb snacks such as cheese, nuts, hard-boiled eggs, or vegetables with dip to keep hunger at bay between meals.

8. *Monitor Portion Sizes:* Pay attention to portion sizes to ensure you're not overeating, even with low-carb foods. While the Atkins diet doesn't typically require strict calorie counting, portion control is still important for weight management.

Breakfast Recipes

Sausage and Mushroom Scramble

Cooking Time: 15 minutes

Servings: 2

Ingredients:

- 4 large eggs
- 4 oz (about 113g) sausage, sliced or crumbled
- 1 cup sliced mushrooms
- ¼ cup diced onion
- 2 tbsp olive oil
- Salt and pepper to taste

Optional: shredded cheese for topping (ensure it fits your Atkins phase)

Instructions:

1. Heat 1 tablespoon of olive oil in a
    skillet over medium heat.

2. Add the sausage slices or crumbles to
    the skillet and cook until browned and
    cooked through, about 5-7 minutes.
    Remove the sausage from the skillet
    and set aside.

3. In the same skillet, add the remaining
    tablespoon of olive oil and sauté the
    onions and mushrooms until softened
    and slightly browned, about 5 minutes.

4. While the onions and mushrooms are
    cooking, crack the eggs into a bowl
    and beat them lightly.

5. Once the mushrooms and onions are
    cooked, add the beaten eggs to the
    skillet, stirring gently to scramble.

6. Cook the eggs until they are set but still slightly moist, about 2-3 minutes.

7. Return the cooked sausage to the skillet and mix it into the scrambled eggs.

8. Season with salt and pepper to taste.

9. Sprinkle shredded cheese on top of the scramble and let it melt slightly if desired.

10. Serve hot and enjoy!

Chia Seed Pudding

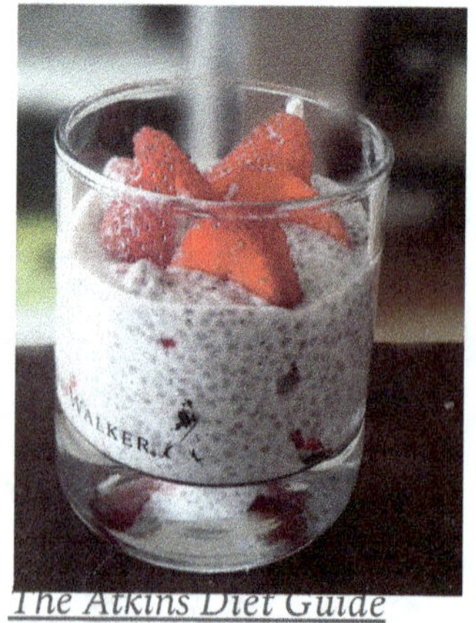

Preparation time: 5 minutes

Chilling time: At least 2 hours

Servings: 2

Ingredients:

- ¼ cup chia seeds
- 1 cup unsweetened almond milk or coconut milk
- ½ teaspoon vanilla extract
- Stevia or other Atkins-friendly sweetener, to taste (optional)
- Fresh berries or nuts for topping (optional)

Instructions:

1. In a mixing bowl, combine chia seeds, almond milk or coconut milk, and vanilla extract. Stir well to ensure chia seeds are evenly distributed.

2. If desired, sweeten the mixture with Atkins-friendly sweetener to taste. Remember to adjust according to your preference.

3. Cover the bowl and refrigerate for at least 2 hours, or overnight, to allow the chia seeds to absorb the liquid and thicken into a pudding-like consistency.

4. After refrigeration, give the pudding a good stir to redistribute the chia seeds.

5. Serve chilled, topped with fresh berries or nuts if desired.

Cauliflower Hash Browns

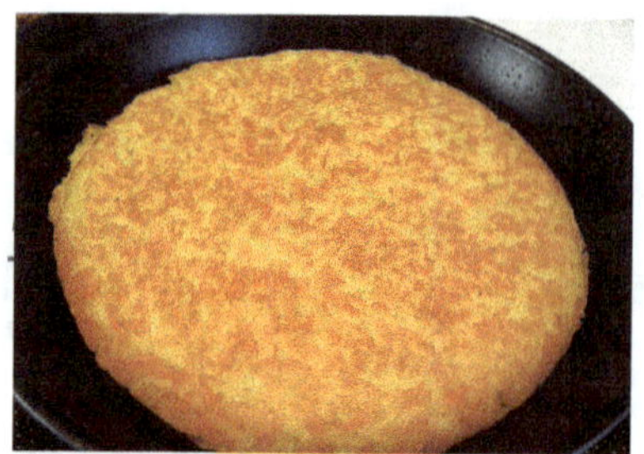

Preparation time: 10 minutes

Baking time: 20-25 minutes

Servings: 3

Ingredients:

- 1 small head of cauliflower, riced (about 2 cups)
- ¼ cup grated parmesan cheese
- ¼ cup almond flour
- 1 egg
- ½ teaspoon garlic powder
- ½ teaspoon onion powder
- Salt and pepper to taste
- Cooking oil or cooking spray

Instructions:

1. Preheat your oven to 400°F (200°C). Line a baking sheet with parchment

paper or lightly grease it with cooking oil or cooking spray.

2. In a large mixing bowl, combine the riced cauliflower, grated parmesan cheese, almond flour, egg, garlic powder, onion powder, salt, and pepper. Mix until well combined.

3. Take a small handful of the cauliflower mixture and shape it into a patty, forming it into a hash brown shape. Repeat with the remaining mixture, making approximately 4-6 hash brown patties depending on the size you prefer.

4. Place the cauliflower hash brown patties onto the prepared baking sheet.

5. Bake in the preheated oven for 20-25 minutes, or until the edges are golden brown and crispy, flipping halfway through the cooking time for even browning.

6. Once cooked, remove the cauliflower hash browns from the oven and let them cool slightly before serving.

Cheesy Broccoli Frittata

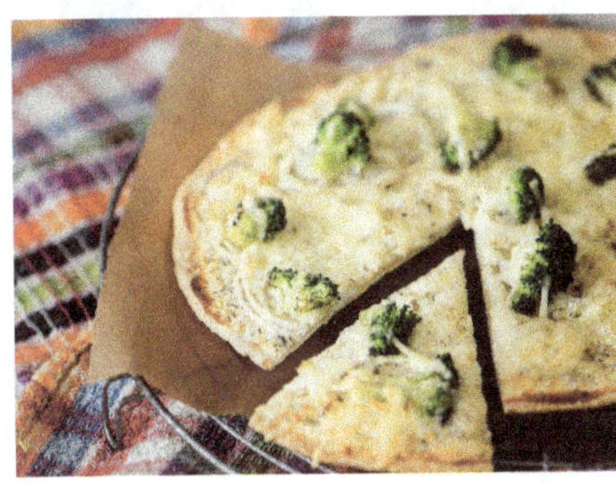

Preparation time: 10 minutes

Cooking time: 8-10 minutes

Servings: 3

Ingredients:

- 6 large eggs
- 1 cup chopped broccoli florets
- ½ cup shredded cheddar cheese
- 2 tablespoons heavy cream
- 1 tablespoon olive oil
- Salt and pepper to taste

Optional: chopped fresh herbs such as parsley or chives for garnish

Instructions:

1. Preheat your oven broiler.
2. In a mixing bowl, whisk together the eggs, heavy cream, salt, and pepper until well combined.
3. Heat olive oil in an oven-safe skillet over medium heat. Add the chopped

broccoli florets and sauté for 2-3 minutes until slightly softened.

4. Pour the egg mixture over the broccoli in the skillet, ensuring the broccoli is evenly distributed.

5. Cook the frittata on the stove for 3-4 minutes, or until the edges start to set.

6. Sprinkle the shredded cheddar cheese evenly over the top of the frittata.

7. Transfer the skillet to the preheated oven broiler and broil for 3-5 minutes, or until the top is golden brown and the center is set.

8. Once cooked, remove the skillet from the oven (remember to use an oven mitt as the handle will be hot) and let it cool slightly.

9. Slice the frittata into wedges, garnish with chopped fresh herbs if desired, and serve hot.

Zucchini and Bacon Muffins

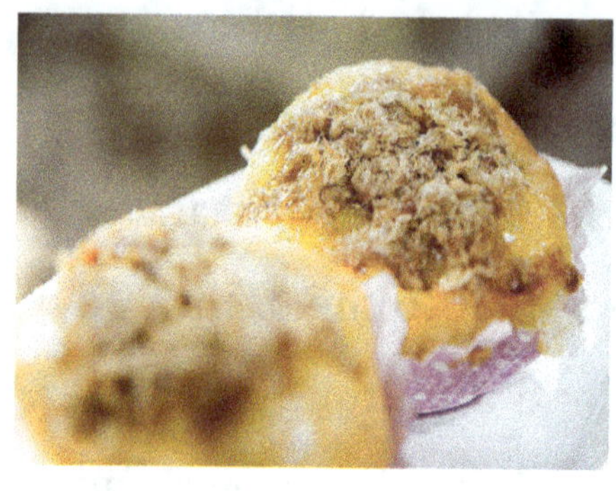

Preparation time: 15 minutes

Baking time: 20-25 minutes

Servings: 6

Ingredients:

- 1 cup almond flour
- 1 teaspoon baking powder
- ½ teaspoon garlic powder

- ½ teaspoon onion powder

- ¼ teaspoon salt

- ¼ teaspoon black pepper

- 2 large eggs

- ¼ cup melted butter or coconut oil

- 1 cup shredded zucchini, excess moisture squeezed out

- ¼ cup cooked bacon, chopped

- ¼ cup shredded cheddar cheese

Instructions:

1. Preheat your oven to 350°F (175°C). Line a muffin tin with paper liners or grease it with cooking oil or cooking spray.

2. In a large mixing bowl, whisk together the almond flour, baking powder,

garlic powder, onion powder, salt, and
black pepper.

3. In a separate bowl, beat the eggs and
   mix in the melted butter or coconut
   oil.

4. Pour the wet ingredients into the dry
   ingredients and stir until well
   combined.

5. Fold in the shredded zucchini,
   chopped bacon, and shredded cheddar
   cheese until evenly distributed
   throughout the batter.

6. Spoon the batter into the prepared
   muffin tin, filling each muffin cup
   about ¾ full.

7. Bake in the preheated oven for 20-25
   minutes, or until the muffins are

golden brown and a toothpick inserted into the center comes out clean.

8. Once cooked, remove the muffins from the oven and let them cool in the muffin tin for a few minutes before transferring them to a wire rack to cool completely.

Keto Smoothie Bowl

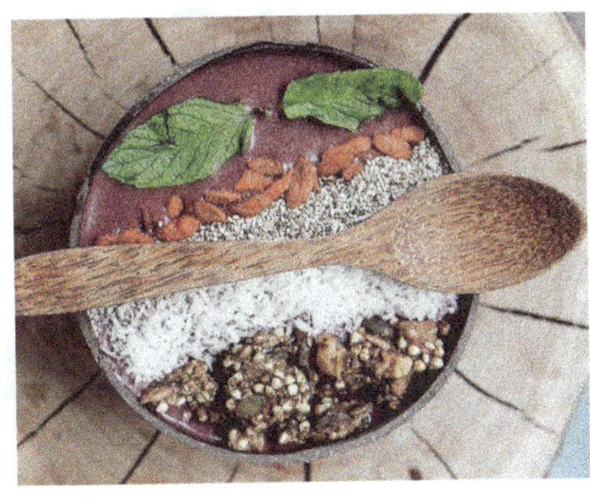

Preparation time: 5 minutes

Servings: 1

Ingredients:

- ½ ripe avocado

- ½ cup unsweetened almond milk or coconut milk
- ¼ cup full-fat Greek yogurt
- ½ cup spinach leaves
- ¼ cup frozen berries (such as raspberries, strawberries, or blueberries)
- 1 tablespoon chia seeds
- 1 tablespoon almond butter or peanut butter (unsweetened)
- ½ teaspoon vanilla extract

Optional toppings: sliced almonds, unsweetened coconut flakes, hemp seeds, additional berries

Instructions:

1. In a blender, combine the ripe avocado, almond milk or coconut milk, Greek yogurt, spinach leaves, frozen berries, chia seeds, almond butter or peanut butter, and vanilla extract.

2. Blend on high speed until smooth and creamy, scraping down the sides of the blender as needed to ensure all ingredients are well incorporated.

3. Once the smoothie mixture is smooth and thick, pour it into a bowl.

4. Top the smoothie bowl with your choice of optional toppings, such as sliced almonds, unsweetened coconut flakes, hemp seeds, and additional berries.

5. Serve immediately and enjoy with a
    spoon.

Low-Carb Breakfast Burrito

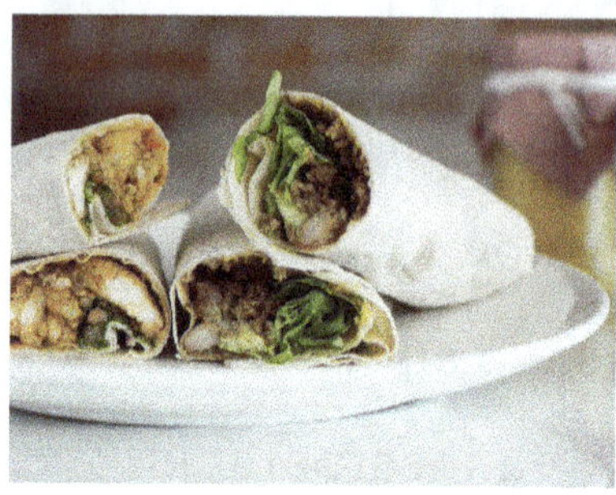

Preparation time:
10 minutes

Cooking time: 10 minutes

Servings: 2

Ingredients:

- 2 large eggs
- 2 slices bacon, cooked until crispy and
  chopped
- ¼ cup diced bell peppers (any color)

- ¼ cup diced onions
- 2 tablespoons shredded cheddar cheese
- 2 large butter lettuce leaves or low-carb tortillas
- Salt and pepper to taste

Optional toppings: avocado slices, salsa, sour cream

Instructions:

1. In a skillet over medium heat, add diced bell peppers and onions. Sauté until they are tender and slightly caramelized, about 5 minutes.
2. While the vegetables are cooking, beat the eggs in a bowl and season with salt and pepper.

3. Push the vegetables to one side of the
   skillet and pour the beaten eggs into
   the empty side. Cook the eggs, stirring
   occasionally, until they are scrambled
   and cooked through.

4. Once the eggs are cooked, remove the
   skillet from heat and stir in the
   chopped bacon and shredded cheddar
   cheese until the cheese is melted.

5. To assemble the breakfast burritos, lay
   out the butter lettuce leaves or
   low-carb tortillas on a flat surface.

6. Spoon the scrambled egg mixture onto
   each lettuce leaf or tortilla, dividing it
   evenly.

7. Add any optional toppings such as
   avocado slices, salsa, or sour cream if
   desired.

8. Roll up the lettuce leaves or tortillas to form burritos, tucking in the sides as you roll.

9. Serve immediately and enjoy your low-carb breakfast burrito!

Avocado Bacon Egg Cups

Preparation time: 10 minutes
Baking time: 15-20 minutes
Servings: 4

Ingredients:
- 2 ripe avocados
- 4 slices bacon
- 4 large eggs
- Salt and pepper to taste

Optional toppings: shredded cheddar cheese, chopped chives

Instructions:

1. Preheat your oven to 375°F (190°C). Grease a muffin tin with cooking spray or line it with silicone muffin liners.

2. Cut the avocados in half lengthwise and remove the pits. Use a spoon to scoop out a little extra avocado flesh from each half to make room for the eggs.

3. Place each avocado half cut-side up in the prepared muffin tin, ensuring they are stable and won't tip over.

4. Wrap each avocado half with a slice of bacon, starting from the top and

wrapping it around the avocado until it overlaps.

5. Crack one egg into each avocado half, making sure to keep the yolk intact.

6. Season each avocado egg cup with salt and pepper to taste.

7. Place the muffin tin in the preheated oven and bake for 15-20 minutes, or until the egg whites are set and the bacon is crispy.

8. Once cooked, remove the avocado bacon egg cups from the oven and let them cool for a few minutes before serving.

9. If desired, sprinkle each avocado egg cup with shredded cheddar cheese and chopped chives before serving.

Lunch Recipes

Zucchini Noodles with Pesto and Chicken

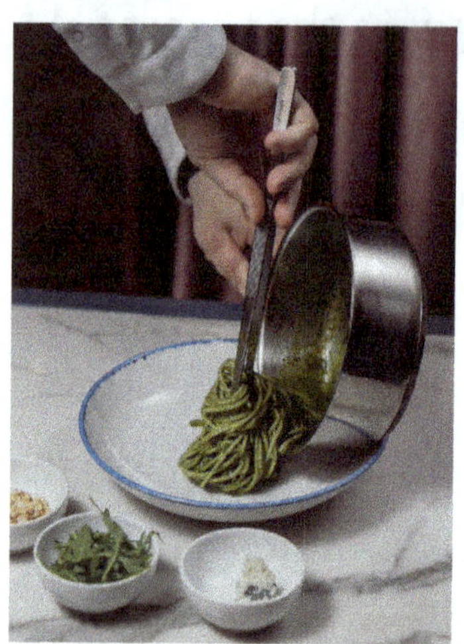

Preparation time: 10 minutes

Cooking time: 15 minutes

Servings: 2

Ingredients:

- 2 medium zucchinis
- 1 tablespoon olive oil

- 2 boneless, skinless chicken breasts, thinly sliced
- Salt and pepper to taste
- ¼ cup prepared pesto sauce

Optional garnish: grated Parmesan cheese, pine nuts, fresh basil leaves

Instructions:

1. Using a spiralizer or vegetable peeler, create zucchini noodles (zoodles) from the zucchinis. Set aside.
2. In a large skillet, heat the olive oil over medium-high heat.
3. Season the thinly sliced chicken breasts with salt and pepper.
4. Add the seasoned chicken slices to the skillet and cook until they are

browned and cooked through, about 5-7 minutes per side.

5. Once the chicken is cooked, remove it from the skillet and set aside.

6. In the same skillet, add the zucchini noodles and cook for 2-3 minutes, tossing occasionally, until they are just tender but still have a slight crunch.

7. Return the cooked chicken to the skillet with the zucchini noodles.

8. Add the prepared pesto sauce to the skillet and toss everything together until the chicken and zucchini noodles are coated evenly with the pesto sauce.

9. Cook for an additional 1-2 minutes, or until everything is heated through.

10. Remove the skillet from heat and divide the zucchini noodles with pesto and chicken among serving plates.

11. If desired, garnish with grated Parmesan cheese, pine nuts, and fresh basil leaves before serving.

Cauliflower Fried Rice

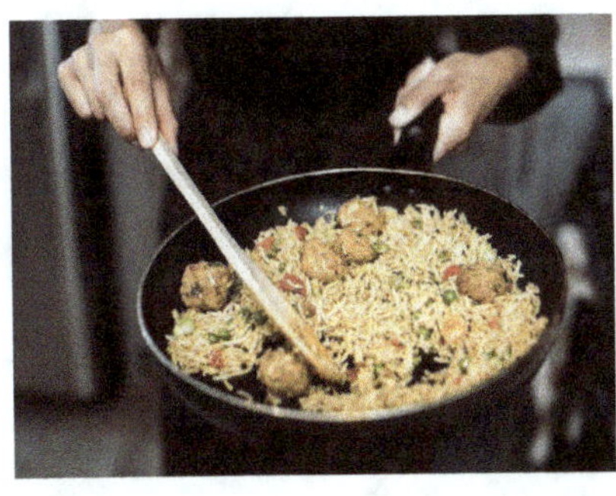

Preparation time: 10 minutes

Cooking time: 10 minutes

Servings: 4

Ingredients:

- 1 medium head of cauliflower

- 2 tablespoons olive oil or coconut oil
- 2 cloves garlic, minced
- 1/2 cup diced carrots
- 1/2 cup diced bell peppers (any color)
- 1/2 cup diced onions
- 2 large eggs, beaten
- 2 tablespoons soy sauce or tamari sauce (for gluten-free option)
- 1 teaspoon sesame oil (optional)
- Salt and pepper to taste

Optional garnish: chopped green onions, sesame seeds.

Instructions:

1. Cut the cauliflower into florets and discard the stems. Place the cauliflower florets in a food processor

and pulse until they resemble rice-like grains. Alternatively, you can grate the cauliflower using a box grater.

2. Heat one tablespoon of olive oil or coconut oil in a large skillet or wok over medium heat.

3. Add the minced garlic to the skillet and sauté for about 30 seconds until fragrant.

4. Add the diced carrots, bell peppers, and onions to the skillet. Cook for 3-4 minutes until the vegetables are tender-crisp.

5. Push the vegetables to one side of the skillet and add the beaten eggs to the empty side. Scramble the eggs until cooked through, then mix them with the cooked vegetables.

6. Push the vegetable and egg mixture to one side of the skillet again, and add the remaining tablespoon of olive oil or coconut oil to the empty side.

7. Add the riced cauliflower to the skillet and stir-fry for 4-5 minutes, or until the cauliflower is tender but not mushy.

8. Stir in the soy sauce or tamari sauce and sesame oil (if using) until everything is well combined.

9. Season with salt and pepper to taste.

10. If desired, garnish with chopped green onions and sesame seeds before serving.

Zucchini Lasagna

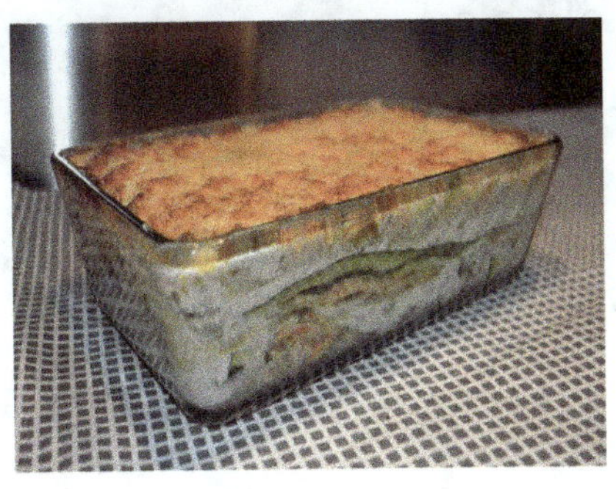

Preparation time:

20 minutes

Baking time:

40-45 minutes

Servings: 6

Ingredients:

- 2 large zucchinis, thinly sliced lengthwise (about 1/4 inch thick)
- 1 pound ground beef or turkey
- 1 small onion, diced
- 2 cloves garlic, minced
- 1 cup marinara sauce (look for a low-carb version)
- 1 cup ricotta cheese
- 1 cup shredded mozzarella cheese
- ¼ cup grated Parmesan cheese

- 1 tablespoon olive oil
- Salt and pepper to taste

Optional: Italian seasoning, chopped fresh basil or parsley for garnish

Instructions:

1. Preheat your oven to 375°F (190°C).
2. In a skillet over medium heat, heat the olive oil. Add the diced onion and minced garlic, and sauté until they are soft and fragrant, about 3-4 minutes.
3. Add the ground beef or turkey to the skillet and cook until browned, breaking it up into smaller pieces with a spatula as it cooks.
4. Once the meat is cooked, stir in the marinara sauce and simmer for a few

minutes. Season with salt, pepper, and Italian seasoning to taste.

5. In a separate bowl, combine the ricotta cheese, half of the shredded mozzarella cheese, and half of the grated Parmesan cheese. Mix well.

6. To assemble the lasagna, spread a thin layer of the meat sauce on the bottom of a baking dish.

7. Layer the thinly sliced zucchini over the meat sauce, covering it completely.

8. Spread a layer of the ricotta cheese mixture over the zucchini slices.

9. Repeat the layers, ending with a layer of meat sauce on top.

10. Sprinkle the remaining shredded mozzarella and grated Parmesan cheese over the top of the lasagna.

11. Cover the baking dish with foil and bake in the preheated oven for 30 minutes.

12. Remove the foil and bake for an additional 10-15 minutes, or until the cheese is melted and bubbly, and the zucchini is tender.

13. Once cooked, remove the lasagna from the oven and let it cool for a few minutes before slicing.

14. Garnish with chopped fresh basil or parsley before serving, if desired.

Stuffed Portobello Mushrooms

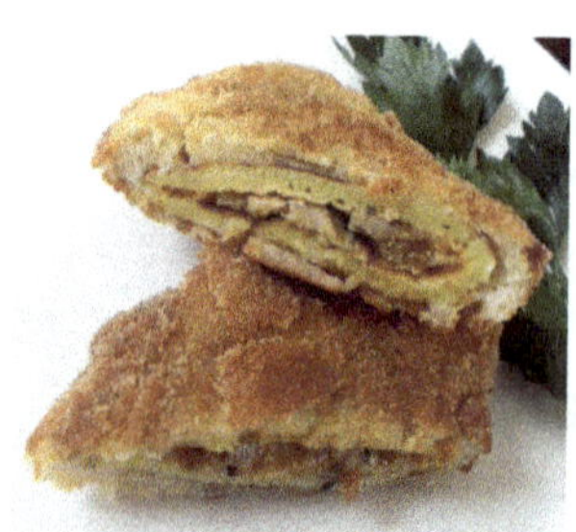

Preparation time: 15 minutes

Baking time: 20-25 minutes

Servings: 4

Ingredients:

- 4 large portobello mushrooms, stems removed
- 1 tablespoon olive oil
- ½ pound ground sausage or ground turkey
- ¼ cup diced onions
- 2 cloves garlic, minced
- ½ cup diced bell peppers (any color)
- 1 cup fresh spinach, chopped
- ½ cup shredded mozzarella cheese
- ¼ cup grated Parmesan cheese
- Salt and pepper to taste

Instructions:

1. Preheat your oven to 375°F (190°C).

2. Clean the portobello mushrooms and
    remove the stems. Place the
    mushrooms on a baking sheet.

3. In a skillet over medium heat, heat the
    olive oil. Add the ground sausage or
    turkey and cook until browned.

4. Add the diced onions, minced garlic,
    and diced bell peppers to the skillet.
    Sauté until the vegetables are
    softened.

5. Stir in the chopped spinach and cook
    until wilted.

6. Season the mixture with salt and
    pepper to taste.

7. Fill each portobello mushroom cap
    with the sausage and vegetable
    mixture.

8. Top each stuffed mushroom with a mixture of shredded mozzarella and grated Parmesan cheese.
9. Bake in the preheated oven for 20-25 minutes, or until the mushrooms are tender and the cheese is melted and golden brown.
10. Garnish with chopped fresh herbs before serving if desired.

Beef and Broccoli Stir-Fry

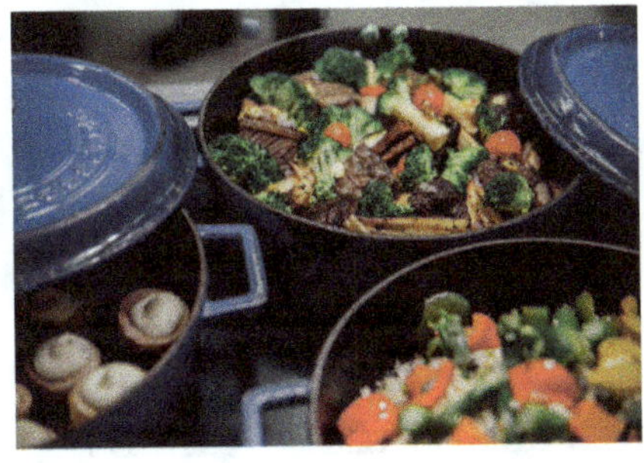

Preparation time: 10 minutes

Cooking time: 10 minutes

Servings: 4

Ingredients:

- 1 pound flank steak, thinly sliced against the grain
- 2 tablespoons soy sauce or tamari sauce (for gluten-free option)
- 1 tablespoon olive oil
- 2 cloves garlic, minced
- 1 teaspoon grated ginger
- 2 cups broccoli florets
- ¼ cup beef broth or water
- Salt and pepper to taste

Instructions:

1. In a bowl, marinate the thinly sliced flank steak with soy sauce or tamari sauce for about 15-20 minutes.

2. Heat olive oil in a large skillet or wok over medium-high heat.

3. Add the minced garlic and grated ginger to the skillet, and sauté for about 30 seconds until fragrant.

4. Add the marinated flank steak to the skillet and stir-fry for 2-3 minutes until browned on all sides.

5. Add the broccoli florets to the skillet and stir-fry for another 2-3 minutes until they are tender-crisp.

6. Pour the beef broth or water into the skillet to deglaze the pan, scraping up any browned bits from the bottom.

7. Continue to cook for another 2-3 minutes until the sauce has thickened slightly and the beef and broccoli are cooked through.

8. Season with salt and pepper to taste.

9. Garnish with sliced green onions and
   sesame seeds before serving if desired.

Low-Carb Chicken Alfredo

Preparation time: 10 minutes
Cooking time: 20 minutes
Servings: 3

Ingredients:

- 2 boneless, skinless chicken breasts
- Salt and pepper to taste
- 1 tablespoon olive oil
- 2 cloves garlic, minced
- 1 cup heavy cream
- ½ cup grated Parmesan cheese
- ¼ teaspoon garlic powder

- ¼ teaspoon onion powder

- ¼ teaspoon dried oregano

- ¼ teaspoon dried basil

- ¼ teaspoon dried thyme

- ¼ teaspoon black pepper

- 2 cups cooked low-carb pasta or zucchini noodles (zoodles)

Instructions:

1. Season the chicken breasts with salt and pepper on both sides.

2. In a skillet over medium-high heat, heat the olive oil. Add the seasoned chicken breasts and cook until they are browned on both sides and cooked through, about 6-8 minutes per side depending on thickness. Remove the chicken from the skillet and set aside.

3. In the same skillet, add the minced
    garlic and sauté for about 30 seconds
    until fragrant.

4. Reduce the heat to medium and pour
    in the heavy cream, stirring to
    combine with the garlic.

5. Add the grated Parmesan cheese,
    garlic powder, onion powder, dried
    oregano, dried basil, dried thyme, and
    black pepper to the skillet. Stir until
    the cheese is melted and the sauce is
    smooth and creamy.

6. Slice the cooked chicken breasts into
    thin strips and return them to the
    skillet, stirring to coat with the
    Alfredo sauce.

7. Cook for an additional 2-3 minutes
    until the chicken is heated through.

8. Add the cooked low-carb pasta or zucchini noodles (zoodles) to the skillet and toss until they are coated evenly with the Alfredo sauce.

9. Cook for another 1-2 minutes until everything is heated through.

10. You can garnish with chopped fresh parsley and grated Parmesan cheese before serving if desired.

Spinach and Bacon Quiche

Preparation time: 15 minutes

Baking time: 35-40 minutes

Servings: 6

Ingredients:

- 1 premade low-carb pie crust (or use a crustless option)
- 6 slices bacon, cooked until crispy and crumbled
- 1 cup fresh spinach, chopped
- ½ cup shredded cheddar cheese
- 4 large eggs
- 1 cup heavy cream or half-and-half
- ¼ teaspoon garlic powder
- Salt and pepper to taste
- Optional: chopped green onions for garnish

Instructions:

1. Preheat your oven to 375°F (190°C). If using a premade pie crust, place it in a pie dish and set aside.

2. In a skillet over medium heat, cook the bacon until crispy. Remove the bacon from the skillet and place it on a paper towel-lined plate to drain excess grease. Once cooled, crumble the bacon into small pieces.

3. In the same skillet, add the chopped spinach and cook until wilted, about 2-3 minutes. Remove from heat and set aside.

4. In a mixing bowl, whisk together the eggs, heavy cream or half-and-half, garlic powder, salt, and pepper until well combined.

5. Spread the crumbled bacon and cooked spinach evenly over the bottom of the pie crust.

6. Sprinkle the shredded cheddar cheese
    over the top of the bacon and spinach.

7. Pour the egg mixture over the bacon,
    spinach, and cheese in the pie crust,
    ensuring it is evenly distributed.

8. Garnish with chopped green onions
    on top (optional)

9. Place the quiche in the preheated oven
    and bake for 35-40 minutes, or until
    the center is set and the top is golden
    brown.

10. Once cooked, remove the quiche from
    the oven and let it cool for a few
    minutes before slicing.

Steak and Veggie Stir-Fry

Preparation time: 15 minutes

Cooking time: 10 minutes

Servings: 4

Ingredients:

- 1 pound steak (such as sirloin or flank steak), thinly sliced
- 2 tablespoons soy sauce or tamari sauce (for gluten-free option)
- 1 tablespoon olive oil
- 2 cloves garlic, minced
- 1 teaspoon grated ginger
- 2 cups mixed vegetables (such as bell peppers, broccoli, snap peas, carrots), sliced or chopped
- Salt and pepper to taste.

Instructions:

1. In a bowl, marinate the thinly sliced
   steak with soy sauce or tamari sauce
   for about 15-20 minutes.

2. Heat olive oil in a large skillet or wok
   over medium-high heat.

3. Add the minced garlic and grated
   ginger to the skillet, and sauté for
   about 30 seconds until fragrant.

4. Add the marinated steak slices to the
   skillet and stir-fry for 2-3 minutes
   until browned on all sides. Remove the
   steak from the skillet and set aside.

5. In the same skillet, add the mixed
   vegetables and stir-fry for 3-4 minutes
   until they are tender-crisp.

6. Return the cooked steak to the skillet
   with the vegetables, and toss

everything together until heated
through.

7. Season with salt and pepper to taste.

8. Garnish with sliced green onions and
   sesame seeds before serving (optional).

Spinach and Feta Stuffed Chicken Breast

Cooking Time: 25-30 minutes
Servings: 4

Ingredients:

- 4 boneless, skinless chicken breasts

- 1 cup chopped spinach (fresh or frozen, thawed and drained)
- ½ cup crumbled feta cheese
- 2 cloves garlic, minced
- 1 tablespoon olive oil
- Salt and pepper to taste
- Toothpicks or kitchen twine

Instructions:

1. Preheat your oven to 375°F (190°C).
2. In a small skillet, heat olive oil over medium heat. Add minced garlic and sauté until fragrant, about 1-2 minutes. Add chopped spinach and cook until wilted, about 2-3 minutes. Remove from heat and let cool slightly.

3. Meanwhile, using a sharp knife, make
   a horizontal slit along the side of each
   chicken breast to form a pocket. Be
   careful not to cut all the way through.

4. In a mixing bowl, combine the cooked
   spinach, feta cheese, salt, and pepper.
   Mix well.

5. Stuff each chicken breast with the
   spinach and feta mixture, using
   toothpicks or kitchen twine to secure
   the opening and hold the stuffing in
   place.

6. Place the stuffed chicken breasts in a
   baking dish lightly coated with
   cooking spray or lined with
   parchment paper.

7. Bake in the preheated oven for 25-30
   minutes, or until the chicken is

cooked through and no longer pink in the center, and the juices run clear.

8. Once cooked, remove the toothpicks or twine before serving.

Stuffed Bell Peppers with Ground Turkey

Cooking Time: 25-30 minutes
Servings: 4 (2 stuffed pepper halves per serving)

Ingredients:

- 4 large bell peppers (any color), halved and seeds removed
- 1 pound ground turkey
- 1 small onion, diced
- 2 cloves garlic, minced
- 1 cup cauliflower rice (fresh or frozen)

- 1 can (14.5 ounces) diced tomatoes, drained
- 1 teaspoon dried oregano
- 1 teaspoon dried basil
- Salt and pepper to taste
- 1 cup shredded mozzarella cheese (optional, for topping)
- Fresh parsley, chopped, for garnish (optional)

Instructions:

1. Preheat your oven to 375°F (190°C).
2. Place the bell pepper halves in a baking dish, cut side up, and set aside.
3. In a large skillet, cook the ground turkey over medium heat until browned and no longer pink. Break up the turkey with a spatula as it cooks.

4. Add diced onion and minced garlic to the skillet with the cooked turkey. Cook for 2-3 minutes, until the onions are translucent and fragrant.

5. Stir in cauliflower rice, diced tomatoes, dried oregano, dried basil, salt, and pepper. Cook for another 5 minutes, allowing the flavors to meld together.

6. Spoon the turkey mixture evenly into the halved bell peppers, pressing down gently to pack the filling.

7. If desired, sprinkle shredded mozzarella cheese over the stuffed peppers.

8. Cover the baking dish with foil and bake in the preheated oven for 25-30

minutes, or until the peppers are tender.

9. Remove the foil and bake for an additional 5 minutes, or until the cheese is melted and bubbly.

10. Garnish with chopped parsley before serving, if desired.

Low-Carb Beef Chili

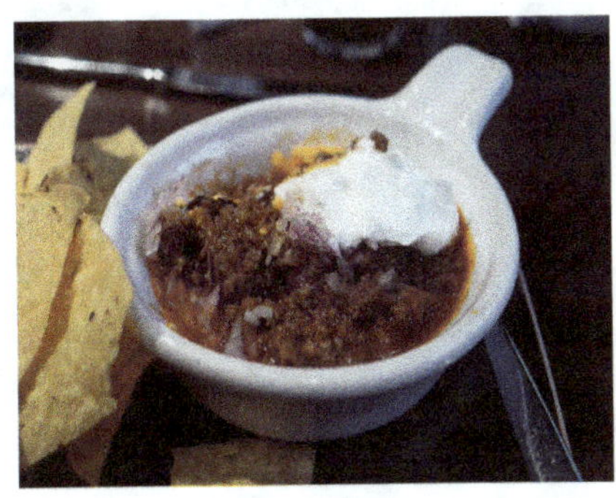

Cooking Time:
20-25 minutes
Servings: 4-6

Ingredients:

- 1 pound lean ground beef

- 1 small onion, diced
- 2 cloves garlic, minced
- 1 bell pepper, diced (any color)
- 1 can (14.5 ounces) diced tomatoes, undrained
- 1 can (6 ounces) tomato paste
- 1 cup beef broth
- 1 tablespoon chili powder
- 1 teaspoon ground cumin
- ½ teaspoon paprika
- ½ teaspoon dried oregano
- Salt and pepper to taste

Optional toppings: shredded cheddar cheese, sour cream, chopped green onions

Instructions:

1. In a large pot or Dutch oven, cook the ground beef over medium heat until browned and no longer pink. Drain any excess fat.

2. Add diced onion, minced garlic, and diced bell pepper to the pot with the cooked beef. Cook for 2-3 minutes, until the vegetables are softened.

3. Stir in diced tomatoes, tomato paste, beef broth, chili powder, ground cumin, paprika, dried oregano, salt, and pepper.

4. Bring the chili to a simmer, then reduce the heat to low. Cover and let it simmer for 20-25 minutes, stirring occasionally to prevent sticking.

5. Taste and adjust seasonings if needed. If the chili is too thick, you can add

more beef broth to reach your desired consistency.

6. Serve the low-carb beef chili hot, topped with shredded cheddar cheese, sour cream, and chopped green onions if desired.

Salmon with Avocado Salsa

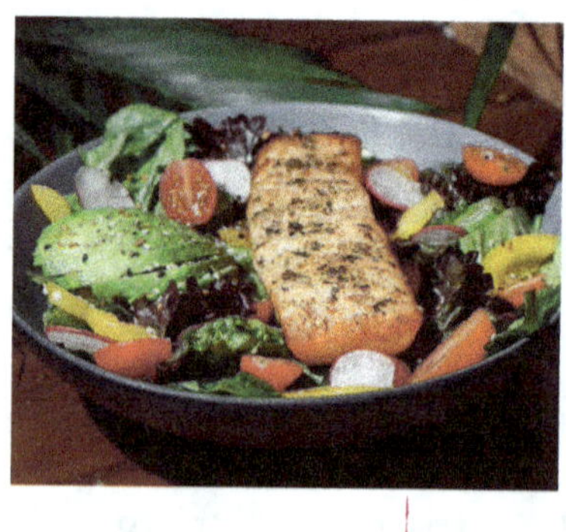

Cooking Time:
8-10 minutes
Servings: 4

Ingredients:

- 4 salmon filets (about 6 ounces each)
- 1 tablespoon olive oil

- Salt and pepper to taste
- For the Avocado Salsa:
    - 2 ripe avocados, diced
    - 1 small tomato, diced
    - ¼ cup red onion, finely chopped
    - 1 jalapeño, seeded and finely chopped
    - Juice of 1 lime
    - 2 tablespoons chopped fresh cilantro
    - Salt and pepper to taste

Instructions:

1. Preheat your grill or grill pan to medium-high heat.
2. Rub the salmon filets with olive oil and season with salt and pepper.

3. Place the salmon filets on the grill, skin side down, and cook for 4-5 minutes per side, or until the fish is cooked through and easily flakes with a fork. Cooking time may vary depending on the thickness of the filets.

4. While the salmon is cooking, prepare the avocado salsa. In a mixing bowl, combine diced avocados, diced tomato, chopped red onion, chopped jalapeño, lime juice, chopped cilantro, salt, and pepper. Gently toss to combine.

5. Once the salmon is cooked, remove it from the grill and transfer it to a serving platter or individual plates.

6. Top the grilled salmon filets with the avocado salsa, dividing it evenly among the filets.

7. Serve immediately, garnished with additional cilantro and lime wedges if desired.

Chicken and Vegetable Kebabs

Cooking Time: 8-10 minutes
Servings: 4

Ingredients:

- 1 pound boneless, skinless chicken breasts, cut into 1-inch cubes
- 1 red bell pepper, cut into 1-inch pieces

- 1 yellow bell pepper, cut into 1-inch pieces
- 1 red onion, cut into 1-inch pieces
- 1 zucchini, sliced into rounds
- 8-10 cherry tomatoes
- 2 tablespoons olive oil
- 2 cloves garlic, minced
- 1 teaspoon dried oregano
- 1 teaspoon dried thyme
- Salt and pepper to taste
- Wooden or metal skewers

Instructions:

1. If you're using wooden skewers, soak them in water for at least 30 minutes to prevent burning while grilling.
2. In a large mixing bowl, combine chicken cubes, bell peppers, red onion,

zucchini, cherry tomatoes, olive oil, minced garlic, dried oregano, dried thyme, salt, and pepper. Toss until the chicken and vegetables are evenly coated with the seasonings.

3. Thread the marinated chicken and vegetables onto the skewers, alternating between the different ingredients.

4. Preheat your grill or grill pan to medium-high heat.

5. Place the skewers on the grill and cook for 8-10 minutes, turning occasionally, until the chicken is cooked through and the vegetables are tender and slightly charred.

6. Once cooked, remove the kebabs from the grill and transfer them to a serving platter.

7. Serve the chicken and vegetable kebabs hot, with your favorite low-carb dipping sauce or alongside a side salad.

Satisfying Soups and Salads

Spicy Sausage and Kale Soup

Cooking Time: 30 minutes

Servings: 4-6

Ingredients:

- 1 lb spicy Italian sausage, casings removed
- 1 onion, chopped
- 3 cloves garlic, minced
- 4 cups chicken broth
- 1 can diced tomatoes (14.5 oz)
- 1 bunch kale, stems removed and leaves chopped
- 1 teaspoon Italian seasoning
- Salt and pepper to taste
- Crushed red pepper flakes (optional, for extra heat)
- Olive oil for cooking

Instructions:

1. Heat a large pot over medium heat and add a drizzle of olive oil.

2. Add the sausage to the pot, breaking it up with a spoon, and cook until browned and cooked through.

3. Remove the cooked sausage from the pot and set aside.

4. In the same pot, add the chopped onion and cook until softened, about 5 minutes.

5. Add the minced garlic and cook for an additional minute until fragrant.

6. Pour in the chicken broth and diced tomatoes, scraping up any browned bits from the bottom of the pot.

7. Stir in the Italian seasoning, salt, pepper, and crushed red pepper flakes if using.

8. Bring the soup to a simmer, then add the chopped kale.

9. Simmer for about 10-15 minutes until the kale is tender.

10. Return the cooked sausage to the pot and heat through.

11. Taste and adjust seasoning if necessary.

12. Serve hot and enjoy!

Creamy Broccoli Soup

Cooking Time: 30 minutes

Servings: 4-6

Ingredients:

- 1 lb broccoli florets, fresh or frozen
- 1 onion, chopped
- 2 cloves garlic, minced
- 4 cups chicken broth

- 1 cup heavy cream
- 2 tablespoons butter
- Salt and pepper to taste
- Olive oil for cooking

Instructions:

1. In a large pot, heat a drizzle of olive oil over medium heat.
2. Add the chopped onion and cook until softened, about 5 minutes.
3. Add the minced garlic and cook for an additional minute until fragrant.
4. Add the broccoli florets to the pot and pour in the chicken broth.
5. Bring the broth to a simmer and cook until the broccoli is tender, about 10-15 minutes.

6. Once the broccoli is tender, remove the pot from the heat and use an immersion blender to blend the soup until smooth. If you don't have an immersion blender, carefully transfer the soup in batches to a blender and blend until smooth, then return it to the pot.

7. Place the pot back on the stove over low heat.

8. Stir in the heavy cream and butter until well combined.

9. Season the soup with salt and pepper to taste.

10. Simmer the soup for an additional 5 minutes to allow the flavors to meld together.

11. Taste and adjust seasoning if necessary.
12. Serve hot and enjoy!

Tomato Basil Soup

Cooking Time: 30 minutes
Servings: 4-6

Ingredients:

- 2 tablespoons olive oil
- 1 onion, chopped
- 2 cloves garlic, minced
- 2 cans diced tomatoes (14.5 oz each), undrained
- 2 cups chicken broth
- ½ cup heavy cream
- ¼ cup fresh basil leaves, chopped

- Salt and pepper to taste

Instructions:

1. Heat the olive oil in a large pot over medium heat.
2. Add the chopped onion and cook until softened, about 5 minutes.
3. Add the minced garlic and cook for another minute until fragrant.
4. Pour in the diced tomatoes with their juices and the chicken broth.
5. Bring the mixture to a simmer and let it cook for about 10-15 minutes.
6. Once the soup has simmered and the flavors have melded, remove it from the heat.
7. Use an immersion blender to blend the soup until smooth. If you don't

have an immersion blender, carefully transfer the soup in batches to a blender and blend until smooth, then return it to the pot.

8. Place the pot back on the stove over low heat.

9. Stir in the heavy cream and chopped basil.

10. Season the soup with salt and pepper to taste.

11. Simmer the soup for an additional 5 minutes to heat through and allow the flavors to come together.

12. Taste and adjust seasoning if necessary.

13. Serve hot, garnished with additional fresh basil leaves if desired.

Thai Coconut Soup

Cooking Time: 25 minutes

Servings: 4-6

Ingredients:

- 1 tablespoon coconut oil
- 1 tablespoon grated ginger
- 2 cloves garlic, minced
- 2 stalks lemongrass, outer layers removed and cut into 2-inch pieces
- 3 cups chicken broth
- 1 can (13.5 oz) full-fat coconut milk
- 2 tablespoons fish sauce
- 1 tablespoon lime juice
- 1 teaspoon chili paste (adjust to taste)
- 1 cup sliced mushrooms
- 1 cup shredded cooked chicken breast

- 1 red bell pepper, thinly sliced
- Salt and pepper to taste
- Fresh cilantro leaves for garnish

Instructions:

1. In a large pot, heat coconut oil over medium heat.

2. Add grated ginger and minced garlic, sauté for about 1 minute until fragrant.

3. Add lemongrass pieces and chicken broth to the pot. Bring to a simmer and let it cook for 10 minutes to infuse the flavors.

4. Stir in coconut milk, fish sauce, lime juice, and chili paste. Simmer for another 5 minutes.

5. Add sliced mushrooms, shredded chicken, and sliced red bell pepper to the pot. Cook for 5-7 minutes until vegetables are tender.

6. Season with salt and pepper to taste.

7. Remove lemongrass pieces from the soup.

8. Serve hot, garnished with fresh cilantro leaves.

Grilled Chicken Caesar Salad

Cooking Time: 15-20 minutes
Servings: 2-4

Ingredients:

- 2 boneless, skinless chicken breasts
- Salt and black pepper to taste

- 1 tablespoon olive oil
- 1 head romaine lettuce, washed and chopped
- ½ cup grated Parmesan cheese
- Caesar salad dressing (store-bought or homemade, low-carb)

Optional toppings: cherry tomatoes, cucumber slices, olives

Instructions:

1. Preheat your grill to medium-high heat.
2. Season the chicken breasts with salt and pepper on both sides.
3. Drizzle olive oil over the chicken breasts.

4. Place the chicken breasts on the preheated grill and cook for 6-8 minutes per side, or until cooked through and no longer pink in the center. Cooking time may vary depending on the thickness of the chicken breasts.

5. Once the chicken is cooked, remove it from the grill and let it rest for a few minutes before slicing it into strips.

6. In a large bowl, toss the chopped romaine lettuce with grated Parmesan cheese.

7. Add the grilled chicken strips on top of the lettuce.

8. Drizzle Caesar salad dressing over the salad according to your preference and toss to coat evenly.

9. Add any optional toppings such as cherry tomatoes, cucumber slices, or olives.

10. Serve immediately and enjoy!

Asian Cucumber Salad

Cooking Time: 30 minutes (mostly marinating time)

Servings: 4-6

Ingredients:

- 2 large cucumbers, thinly sliced
- ¼ cup rice vinegar
- 2 tablespoons soy sauce (or tamari for gluten-free)
- 1 tablespoon sesame oil

- 1 tablespoon granulated sugar substitute (e.g., erythritol or stevia)
- 1 teaspoon grated ginger
- 1 clove garlic, minced
- 1 tablespoon toasted sesame seeds

Optional: chopped green onions or cilantro for garnish

Instructions:

1. In a small bowl, whisk together rice vinegar, soy sauce, sesame oil, sugar substitute, grated ginger, and minced garlic until well combined.
2. Place the thinly sliced cucumbers in a large bowl.
3. Pour the prepared dressing over the cucumbers and toss until evenly coated.

4. Cover the bowl and refrigerate for at least 30 minutes to allow the flavors to meld together.

5. Before serving, sprinkle toasted sesame seeds over the salad and garnish with chopped green onions or cilantro if desired.

6. Serve chilled and enjoy!

Broccoli Bacon Salad

Cooking Time: 15 minutes (mostly assembly and refrigeration time)
Servings: 4-6

Ingredients:

- 4 cups broccoli florets, chopped into bite-sized pieces

- 6 slices bacon, cooked and crumbled
- ¼ cup red onion, finely chopped
- ½ cup mayonnaise (sugar-free or homemade for Atkins diet)
- 2 tablespoons apple cider vinegar
- 1 tablespoon granulated sugar substitute (e.g., erythritol or stevia)
- Salt and black pepper to taste

Optional: shredded cheddar cheese, sunflower seeds, chopped pecans

Instructions:

1. In a large bowl, combine the chopped broccoli florets, crumbled bacon, and chopped red onion.
2. In a small bowl, whisk together mayonnaise, apple cider vinegar, and

granulated sugar substitute until smooth.

3. Pour the dressing over the broccoli mixture and toss until everything is evenly coated.

4. Season with salt and black pepper to taste.

5. Cover the bowl and refrigerate for at least 30 minutes to allow the flavors to meld together.

6. Before serving, give the salad a final toss.

7. If desired, sprinkle shredded cheddar cheese, sunflower seeds, or chopped pecans over the top as garnish.

8. Serve chilled and enjoy!

Keto Cheesecake

Cooking Time: 1 hour 10 minutes (including cooling time)

Servings: 12 slices

Ingredients:

- 2 cups almond flour
- ¼ cup powdered erythritol or monk fruit sweetener
- ½ cup melted butter
- 3 (8-ounce) packages cream cheese, softened
- ¾ cup powdered erythritol or monk fruit sweetener
- 3 large eggs
- 1 teaspoon vanilla extract

- ¼ cup sour cream

- ¼ cup heavy cream

Instructions:

1. Preheat your oven to 325°F (160°C). Grease a 9-inch springform pan with butter or line it with parchment paper.

2. In a mixing bowl, combine almond flour, ¼ cup powdered erythritol or monk fruit sweetener, and melted butter. Press the mixture evenly into the bottom of the prepared springform pan to form the crust. Bake for 10-12 minutes, or until lightly golden. Remove from the oven and let it cool while preparing the filling.

3. In a large mixing bowl, beat the softened cream cheese and 3/4 cup

powdered erythritol or monk fruit sweetener until smooth and creamy.

4. Add eggs, one at a time, mixing well after each addition.

5. Stir in vanilla extract, sour cream, and heavy cream until well combined.

6. Pour the cheesecake filling over the cooled crust, spreading it out evenly.

7. Bake in the preheated oven for 45-50 minutes, or until the center is almost set but still slightly jiggly.

8. Turn off the oven and let the cheesecake cool in the oven with the door closed for 1 hour.

9. Remove the cheesecake from the oven and let it cool completely on a wire rack. Once cooled, refrigerate for at

least 4 hours or overnight before serving.

10. Serve chilled and enjoy!

Chocolate Avocado Mousse

Cooking Time: 10 minutes

Servings: 4

Ingredients:

- 2 ripe avocados
- ¼ cup unsweetened cocoa powder
- ¼ cup powdered erythritol or monk fruit sweetener
- 1 teaspoon vanilla extract
- ¼ cup unsweetened almond milk or coconut milk

Optional toppings: whipped cream, shaved dark chocolate, chopped nuts

Instructions:

1. Cut the avocados in half and remove the pits. Scoop out the flesh and place it in a blender or food processor.
2. Add cocoa powder, powdered erythritol or monk fruit sweetener, vanilla extract, and almond milk or coconut milk to the blender.
3. Blend the mixture until smooth and creamy, scraping down the sides of the blender or food processor as needed.
4. Taste the mousse and adjust the sweetness if necessary by adding more powdered erythritol or monk fruit sweetener.

5. Once the mousse is smooth and well combined, transfer it to serving bowls or glasses.

6. Chill the mousse in the refrigerator for at least 30 minutes before serving.

7. Before serving, you can optionally top the mousse with whipped cream, shaved dark chocolate, or chopped nuts for added flavor and texture.

8. Serve chilled and enjoy!

Almond Flour Blueberry Muffins

Cooking Time: 20-25 minutes
Servings: 12 muffins

Ingredients:

- 2 cups almond flour

- ¼ cup powdered erythritol or monk fruit sweetener
- 1 teaspoon baking powder
- ¼ teaspoon salt
- 3 large eggs
- ¼ cup melted coconut oil or butter
- ¼ cup unsweetened almond milk
- 1 teaspoon vanilla extract
- 1 cup fresh or frozen blueberries

Instructions:

1. Preheat your oven to 350°F (175°C). Line a muffin tin with paper liners or grease it with butter or cooking spray.

2. In a large mixing bowl, combine almond flour, powdered erythritol or monk fruit sweetener, baking powder, and salt.

3. In another bowl, whisk together eggs, melted coconut oil or butter, almond milk, and vanilla extract until well combined.

4. Pour the wet ingredients into the dry ingredients and mix until just combined. Be careful not to overmix.

5. Gently fold in the blueberries until evenly distributed throughout the batter.

6. Spoon the batter into the prepared muffin tin, filling each cup about 3/4 full.

7. Bake in the preheated oven for 20-25 minutes, or until the muffins are golden brown and a toothpick inserted into the center comes out clean.

8. Remove the muffins from the oven and let them cool in the pan for 5 minutes before transferring them to a wire rack to cool completely.

9. Once cooled, serve and enjoy!

Strawberry Cream Cheese Fat Bombs

Cooking Time: 1 hour (chilling time)
Servings: 12 fat bombs

Ingredients:

- 4 ounces cream cheese, softened
- 1/4 cup unsalted butter, softened
- 1/4 cup powdered erythritol or monk fruit sweetener
- 1/2 teaspoon vanilla extract
- 1/4 cup diced fresh strawberries

Optional: unsweetened shredded coconut or chopped nuts for coating

Instructions:

1. In a mixing bowl, combine softened cream cheese, softened butter, powdered erythritol or monk fruit sweetener, and vanilla extract. Mix until smooth and creamy.
2. Gently fold in the diced strawberries until evenly distributed throughout the mixture.
3. Line a small baking dish or tray with parchment paper.
4. Using a small cookie scoop or spoon, portion out the cream cheese mixture into small balls and place them on the lined baking dish or tray.

5. Roll each fat bomb in unsweetened shredded coconut or chopped nuts for added flavor and texture (optional).

6. Once all the fat bombs are formed, place the baking dish or tray in the refrigerator to chill for at least 1 hour, or until firm.

7. Once firm, transfer the fat bombs to an airtight container and store them in the refrigerator until ready to serve.

8. Enjoy these strawberry cream cheese fat bombs as a satisfying and delicious keto-friendly snack!

Lemon Coconut Bliss Balls

Cooking Time: 30 minutes (chilling time)
Servings: 12 bliss balls

Ingredients:

- 1 cup almond flour
- ½ cup unsweetened shredded coconut, plus extra for rolling
- ¼ cup powdered erythritol or monk fruit sweetener
- Zest of 1 lemon
- 2 tablespoons fresh lemon juice
- 2 tablespoons melted coconut oil
- ½ teaspoon vanilla extract
- Pinch of salt

Instructions:

1. In a mixing bowl, combine almond flour, shredded coconut, powdered erythritol or monk fruit sweetener,

lemon zest, and a pinch of salt. Mix
well to combine.

2. Add fresh lemon juice, melted coconut
   oil, and vanilla extract to the dry
   ingredients. Mix until a dough forms.
   If the dough is too dry, you can add a
   little more melted coconut oil.

3. Once the dough is well combined, use
   your hands to roll it into small balls,
   about 1 inch in diameter.

4. Place some additional shredded
   coconut on a plate. Roll each bliss ball
   in the shredded coconut until evenly
   coated.

5. Once all the bliss balls are coated,
   place them on a parchment-lined
   baking sheet or plate.

6. Chill the bliss balls in the refrigerator for at least 30 minutes to firm up.

7. Once firm, transfer the lemon coconut bliss balls to an airtight container and store them in the refrigerator until ready to serve.

8. Enjoy these refreshing and satisfying bliss balls as a snack or dessert option on your Atkins diet!

Meat and Seafood Recipes

Keto Meatballs

Cooking Time: 20-25 minutes

Servings: 20 meatballs

Ingredients:

- 1 lb ground beef (preferably lean)
- ¼ cup almond flour
- ¼ cup grated parmesan cheese
- 1 large egg
- 2 cloves garlic, minced
- 1 teaspoon dried oregano
- 1 teaspoon dried basil
- ½ teaspoon salt
- ¼ teaspoon black pepper
- 1 tablespoon olive oil (for cooking)

Instructions:

1. Preheat your oven to 375°F (190°C).

2. In a large mixing bowl, combine ground beef, almond flour, parmesan cheese, egg, minced garlic, oregano, basil, salt, and black pepper. Mix well until all ingredients are evenly incorporated.

3. Shape the mixture into small meatballs, about 1 inch in diameter, and place them on a baking sheet lined with parchment paper.

4. Drizzle the meatballs with olive oil, then bake in the preheated oven for 20-25 minutes, or until they are cooked through and golden brown.

5. Once cooked, remove the meatballs from the oven and let them cool slightly before serving.

Baked Lemon Herb Chicken

Cooking Time: 20-25 minutes

Servings: 4

Ingredients:

- 4 boneless, skinless chicken breasts
- 2 tablespoons olive oil
- 2 cloves garlic, minced
- Zest and juice of 1 lemon
- 1 teaspoon dried thyme
- 1 teaspoon dried rosemary
- 1 teaspoon dried oregano
- Salt and pepper to taste
- Lemon slices for garnish (optional)
- Fresh parsley for garnish (optional)

Instructions:

1. Preheat your oven to 375°F (190°C).

2. In a small bowl, mix together olive oil, minced garlic, lemon zest, lemon juice, thyme, rosemary, oregano, salt, and pepper to create a marinade.

3. Place the chicken breasts in a shallow dish or a resealable plastic bag, and pour the marinade over them, making sure the chicken is evenly coated. Marinate in the refrigerator for at least 30 minutes, or up to overnight for maximum flavor.

4. Once marinated, transfer the chicken breasts to a baking dish lined with parchment paper or lightly greased with olive oil.

5. Bake the chicken in the preheated oven for 25-30 minutes, or until the chicken is cooked through and reaches an internal temperature of 165°F (74°C).

6. Once cooked, remove the chicken from the oven and let it rest for a few minutes before serving.

7. Garnish with lemon slices and fresh parsley if desired before serving.

Grilled Steak with Chimichurri Sauce

Cooking Time: 8-10 minutes

Servings: 4

Ingredients:

- 4 steaks (such as ribeye, sirloin, or flank steak), about 6-8 ounces each
- Salt and pepper to taste
- Olive oil for grilling

For the Chimichurri Sauce:

- 1 cup fresh parsley, finely chopped
- ¼ cup fresh cilantro, finely chopped
- 3 cloves garlic, minced
- 1 shallot, finely chopped
- ¼ cup red wine vinegar
- ½ cup olive oil
- ½ teaspoon dried oregano
- ½ teaspoon red pepper flakes (adjust to taste)
- Salt and pepper to taste

Instructions:

1. Preheat your grill to medium-high heat.

2. Season the steaks generously with salt and pepper on both sides.

3. Brush the steaks with a little olive oil to prevent sticking to the grill.

4. Place the steaks on the preheated grill and cook for about 4-5 minutes per side for medium-rare, or adjust cooking time according to your desired doneness.

5. While the steaks are grilling, prepare the chimichurri sauce. In a small bowl, combine the chopped parsley, cilantro, minced garlic, chopped shallot, red wine vinegar, olive oil, dried oregano,

red pepper flakes, salt, and pepper. Mix well to combine.

6. Once the steaks are cooked to your liking, remove them from the grill and let them rest for a few minutes.

7. Serve the grilled steaks hot, topped with a generous spoonful of chimichurri sauce.

Keto Shrimp Alfredo

Cooking Time: 15 minutes
Servings: 4

Ingredients:

- 1 lb shrimp, peeled and deveined
- 2 tablespoons olive oil
- 4 cloves garlic, minced

- 1 cup heavy cream
- ½ cup grated parmesan cheese
- Salt and pepper to taste
- 12 oz shirataki noodles or zucchini noodles (zoodles)

Instructions:

1. Heat olive oil in a large skillet over medium heat. Add minced garlic and cook for 1-2 minutes until fragrant.
2. Add the shrimp to the skillet and cook for 2-3 minutes on each side until they turn pink and opaque. Remove the shrimp from the skillet and set aside.
3. In the same skillet, pour in the heavy cream and bring it to a simmer. Let it cook for about 2 minutes.

4. Gradually add the grated parmesan cheese to the cream sauce, stirring constantly, until the cheese is melted and the sauce is smooth and creamy.

5. Season the Alfredo sauce with salt and pepper to taste.

6. Return the cooked shrimp to the skillet and stir until they are coated in the Alfredo sauce.

7. Meanwhile, prepare the shirataki noodles or zucchini noodles according to package instructions.

8. Serve the shrimp Alfredo over the cooked noodles.

Crab-Stuffed Mushrooms

Cooking Time: 15-20 minutes

Servings: 4

Ingredients:

- 12 large mushrooms, cleaned and stems removed
- 1 cup lump crabmeat, drained
- ¼ cup cream cheese, softened
- ¼ cup grated parmesan cheese
- 2 cloves garlic, minced
- 2 green onions, finely chopped
- 1 tablespoon fresh parsley, chopped
- ½ teaspoon Old Bay seasoning (optional)
- Salt and pepper to taste
- 1 tablespoon olive oil

Instructions:

1. Preheat your oven to 375°F (190°C).

2. In a mixing bowl, combine the lump crabmeat, softened cream cheese, grated parmesan cheese, minced garlic, chopped green onions, chopped parsley, Old Bay seasoning (if using), salt, and pepper. Mix well until all ingredients are evenly incorporated.

3. Stuff each mushroom cap with a generous amount of the crab meat mixture, pressing it down gently to fill the cavity.

4. Place the stuffed mushrooms on a baking sheet lined with parchment paper.

5. Drizzle the stuffed mushrooms with olive oil.

6. Bake in the preheated oven for 15-20 minutes, or until the mushrooms are tender and the filling is heated through and lightly golden on top.

7. Once cooked, remove the stuffed mushrooms from the oven and let them cool slightly before serving.

Swordfish Steaks with Tomato Basil Relish

Cooking Time: 8-10 minutes

Servings: 4

Ingredients:

- 4 swordfish steaks, about 6 ounces each
- Salt and pepper to taste
- 2 tablespoons olive oil

For the Tomato Basil Relish:

- 2 cups cherry tomatoes, halved
- ¼ cup fresh basil leaves, thinly sliced
- 2 tablespoons balsamic vinegar
- 1 tablespoon olive oil
- 2 cloves garlic, minced
- Salt and pepper to taste

Instructions:

1. Preheat your grill or grill pan to medium-high heat.
2. Season the swordfish steaks generously with salt and pepper on both sides.
3. Drizzle the swordfish steaks with olive oil and rub to coat evenly.

4. Place the swordfish steaks on the preheated grill or grill pan and cook for 4-5 minutes per side, or until the fish is cooked through and has nice grill marks. Cooking time may vary depending on the thickness of the steaks.

5. While the swordfish is cooking, prepare the tomato basil relish. In a small bowl, combine the halved cherry tomatoes, thinly sliced basil leaves, balsamic vinegar, olive oil, minced garlic, salt, and pepper. Toss to coat the tomatoes evenly in the dressing.

6. Once the swordfish steaks are cooked, remove them from the grill and transfer to serving plates.

7. Spoon the tomato basil relish over the top of each swordfish steak.

8. Serve immediately, garnished with additional fresh basil leaves if desired.

Eggplant Bruschetta

Cooking Time: 30 minutes

Servings: 4

Ingredients:

- 1 large eggplant, sliced into 1/2 inch rounds
- 2 tablespoons olive oil

- Salt and pepper to taste
- 2 large tomatoes, diced
- 2 cloves garlic, minced
- ¼ cup fresh basil, chopped
- 2 tablespoons balsamic vinegar
- ¼ cup grated Parmesan cheese (optional)

Instructions:

1. Preheat your oven to 400°F (200°C).

2. Place eggplant slices on a baking sheet and brush both sides with olive oil. Season with salt and pepper.

3. Roast the eggplant slices in the preheated oven for 15-20 minutes, or until they are tender and slightly golden brown.

4. While the eggplant is roasting, prepare the bruschetta topping. In a bowl, mix together diced tomatoes, minced garlic, chopped basil, and balsamic vinegar. Season with salt and pepper to taste.

5. Once the eggplant slices are done, remove them from the oven and let them cool slightly.

6. Top each eggplant slice with a spoonful of the bruschetta mixture.

7. Optionally, sprinkle grated Parmesan cheese on top of each bruschetta.

8. Return the topped eggplant slices to the oven and bake for an additional 5-7 minutes, or until the cheese is melted and bubbly.

9. Serve the eggplant bruschetta warm, garnished with additional basil if desired.

Crispy Prosciutto-Wrapped Asparagus

Cooking Time: 20-25 minutes
Servings: 4

Ingredients:

- 1 bunch asparagus spears, tough ends trimmed
- 8 slices prosciutto
- Olive oil cooking spray
- Salt and pepper to taste
- Lemon wedges for serving (optional)

Instructions:

1. Preheat your oven to 400°F (200°C).

2. Divide the asparagus spears into 8 equal bundles.

3. Take one slice of prosciutto and wrap it tightly around each bundle of asparagus, starting from the bottom and working your way to the top. Repeat with the remaining asparagus and prosciutto slices.

4. Place the prosciutto-wrapped asparagus bundles on a baking sheet lined with parchment paper.

5. Lightly spray the bundles with olive oil cooking spray and season with salt and pepper to taste.

6. Roast the asparagus in the preheated oven for 10-12 minutes, or until the

asparagus is tender and the prosciutto
is crispy.

7. Remove from the oven and let cool for
    a few minutes before serving.

8. Optionally, serve with lemon wedges
    for squeezing over the asparagus
    before eating.

Cheese Crisps

Cooking Time: 10 minutes

Servings: 4

Ingredients:

- 1 cup shredded cheese (cheddar,
  Parmesan, or your choice)

Optional: Herbs or spices of your choice
(such as garlic powder, smoked paprika, or
dried herbs)

Instructions:

1. Preheat your oven to 400°F (200°C)
    and line a baking sheet with
    parchment paper.
2. Place small piles of shredded cheese
    on the prepared baking sheet, leaving
    some space between each pile. Make
    sure the piles are evenly sized.
3. Optionally, sprinkle your choice of
    herbs or spices over the cheese piles
    for added flavor.
4. Bake the cheese piles in the preheated
    oven for 5-7 minutes, or until the

edges are golden brown and the
cheese has melted and crisped up.

5. Remove the baking sheet from the
oven and let the cheese crisps cool for
a few minutes on the pan.

6. Once cooled slightly, carefully transfer
the cheese crisps to a plate or wire
rack to cool completely and crisp up
further.

7. Repeat the process with any
remaining cheese if needed.

8. Serve the cheese crisps as a crunchy
and satisfying snack or appetizer.

Tuna Cucumber Bites

Preparation Time: 15 minutes

Servings: 4

Ingredients:

- 1 large cucumber
- 1 can (5 oz) tuna, drained
- 2 tablespoons mayonnaise
- 1 tablespoon lemon juice
- Salt and pepper to taste

Optional garnish: Fresh dill, parsley, or chives

Instructions:

1. Peel the cucumber and cut it into slices, about 1/4 inch thick.

2. Use a small spoon or a melon baller to
   hollow out the center of each
   cucumber slice, creating a small well
   for the tuna filling. Place the
   hollowed-out cucumber slices on a
   serving platter.

3. In a mixing bowl, combine the drained
   tuna, mayonnaise, and lemon juice.
   Stir until well combined. Season with
   salt and pepper to taste.

4. Spoon a small amount of the tuna
   mixture into each cucumber slice,
   filling the wells.

5. Garnish each cucumber bite with
   fresh dill, parsley, or chives for added
   flavor and presentation (optional).

6. Serve immediately, or refrigerate until
   ready to serve.

Guacamole Deviled Eggs

Preparation Time: 20 minutes

Servings: 4 (2 halves per serving)

Ingredients:

- 4 hard-boiled eggs, peeled and halved lengthwise
- 1 ripe avocado
- 1 tablespoon lime juice
- 1 tablespoon chopped fresh cilantro
- 1/4 teaspoon garlic powder
- Salt and pepper to taste
- Optional garnish: Chopped tomato, diced red onion, sliced jalapeno

Instructions:

1. Slice the hard-boiled eggs in half lengthwise and carefully remove the yolks. Place the egg whites on a serving platter.

2. In a mixing bowl, mash the ripe avocado with a fork until smooth.

3. Add lime juice, chopped cilantro, garlic powder, salt, and pepper to the mashed avocado. Mix until well combined.

4. Spoon the guacamole mixture into the hollowed-out egg whites, dividing it evenly among them.

5. Garnish each guacamole deviled egg with chopped tomato, diced red onion, or sliced jalapeno for added flavor and presentation (optional).

6. Serve immediately, or refrigerate until
    ready to serve.

CHAPTER FIVE

28-DAY MEAL PLAN

Day 1

Breakfast: Chia Seed Pudding

Lunch: Avocado Bacon Egg Cups

Dinner: Steak and Veggie Stir-Fry

Day 2

Breakfast: Keto Smoothie Bowl

Lunch: Lemon Coconut Bliss Balls

Dinner: Zucchini Lasagna

Day 3

Breakfast: Cheesy Broccoli Frittata

Lunch: Salmon with Avocado Salsa

Dinner: Strawberry Cream Cheese Fat Bombs

Day 4

Breakfast: Spinach and Feta Stuffed Chicken Breast

Lunch: Asian Cucumber Salad

Dinner: Eggplant Bruschetta

Day 5

Breakfast: Cauliflower Hash Browns

Lunch: Grilled Chicken Caesar Salad

Dinner: Chicken and Vegetable Kebabs

Day 6

Breakfast: Cauliflower Hash Browns

Lunch: Grilled Chicken Caesar Salad

Dinner: Chicken and Vegetable Kebabs

Breakfast: Sausage and Mushroom Scramble

Lunch: Guacamole Deviled Eggs

Dinner: Tomato Basil Soup

Day 8

Breakfast: Keto Smoothie Bowl

Lunch: Lemon Coconut Bliss Balls

Dinner: Zucchini Lasagna

Day 9

Breakfast: Cheesy Broccoli Frittata

Lunch: Salmon with Avocado Salsa

Dinner: Strawberry Cream Cheese Fat Bombs

Day 10

Breakfast: Beef and Broccoli Stir-Fry

Lunch: Tomato Basil Soup

Dinner: Spinach and Bacon Quiche

Day 11

Breakfast: Sausage and Mushroom Scramble

Lunch: Guacamole Deviled Eggs

Dinner: Tomato Basil Soup

Day 12

Breakfast: Low-Carb Breakfast Burrito

Lunch: Spicy Sausage and Kale Soup

Dinner: Zucchini Lasagna

Day 13

Breakfast: Cheesy Broccoli Frittata

Lunch: Keto Cheesecake

Dinner: Grilled Chicken Caesar Salad

Day 14

Breakfast: Chia Seed Pudding

Lunch: Zucchini Noodles with Pesto and Chicken

Dinner: Broccoli Bacon Salad

Day 15

Breakfast: Cauliflower Hash Browns

Lunch: Grilled Chicken Caesar Salad

Dinner: Chicken and Vegetable Kebabs

Day 16

Breakfast: Low-Carb Breakfast Burrito

Lunch: Chocolate Avocado Mousse

Dinner: Steak and Veggie Stir-Fry

Breakfast: Keto Smoothie Bowl

Lunch: Lemon Coconut Bliss Balls

Dinner: Zucchini Lasagna

Day 18

Breakfast: Cheesy Broccoli Frittata

Lunch: Salmon with Avocado Salsa

Dinner: Strawberry Cream Cheese Fat Bombs

Day 19

Breakfast: Sausage and Mushroom Scramble

Lunch: Guacamole Deviled Eggs

Dinner: Tomato Basil Soup

Day 20

Breakfast: Spinach and Feta Stuffed Chicken Breast

Lunch: Asian Cucumber Salad

Dinner: Eggplant Bruschetta

Day 21

Breakfast: Beef and Broccoli Stir-Fry

Lunch: Tomato Basil Soup

Dinner: Spinach and Bacon Quiche

Day 22

Breakfast: Zucchini and Bacon Muffins

Lunch: Thai Coconut Soup

Dinner: Zucchini Lasagna

Day 23

Breakfast: Keto Smoothie Bowl

Lunch: Cauliflower Fried Rice

Dinner: Chicken and Vegetable Kebabs

Breakfast: Cheesy Broccoli Frittata

Lunch: Beef and Broccoli Stir-Fry

Dinner: Stuffed Bell Peppers with Ground Turkey

Day 25

Breakfast: Low-Carb Breakfast Burrito

Lunch: Guacamole Deviled Eggs

Dinner: Salmon with Avocado Salsa

Day 26

Breakfast: Cauliflower Hash Browns

Lunch: Stuffed Portobello Mushrooms

Dinner: Low-Carb Beef Chili

Day 27

Breakfast: Chia Seed Pudding

Lunch: Avocado Bacon Egg Cups

Dinner: Steak and Veggie Stir-Fry

Day 28

Breakfast: Sausage and Mushroom Scramble

Lunch: Zucchini Noodles with Pesto and Chicken

Dinner: Spinach and Feta Stuffed Chicken Breast

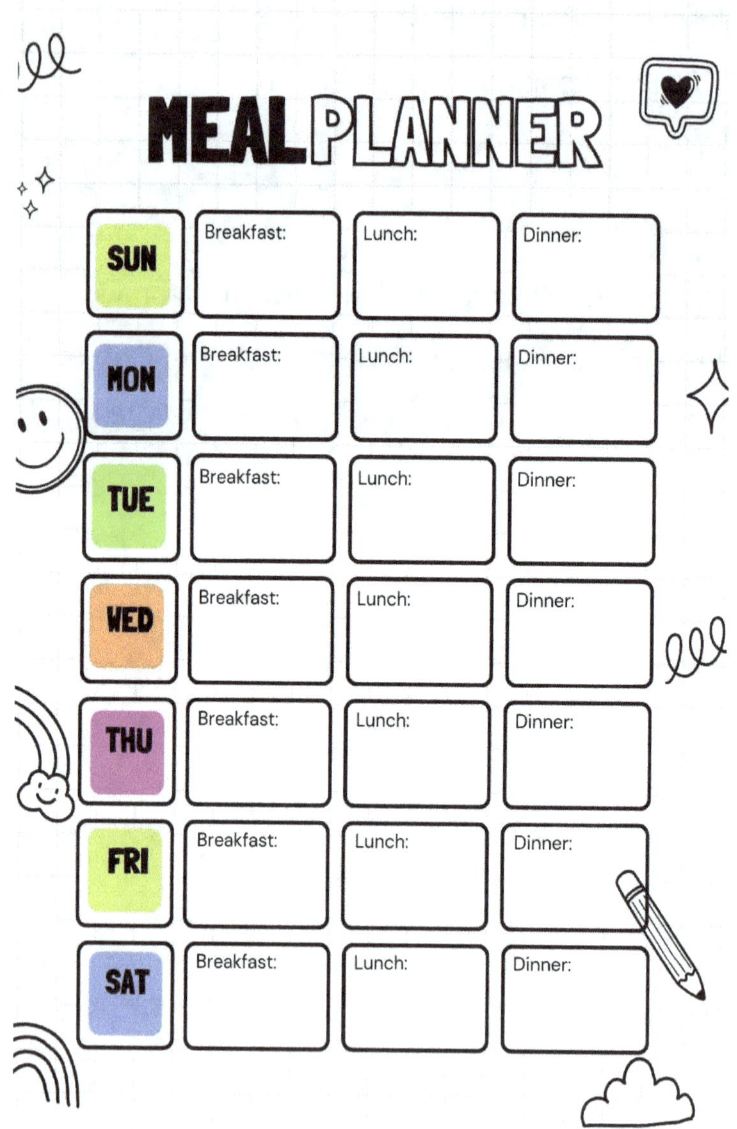

MEAL PLANNER
SUN
Breakfast:
Lunch:
Dinner:
MON
Breakfast:
Lunch:
Dinner:
TUE
Breakfast:
Lunch:
Dinner:
WED
Breakfast:
Lunch:
Dinner:
THU
Breakfast:
Lunch:
Dinner:
FRI
Breakfast:
Lunch:
Dinner:
SAT
Breakfast:
Lunch:
Dinner:

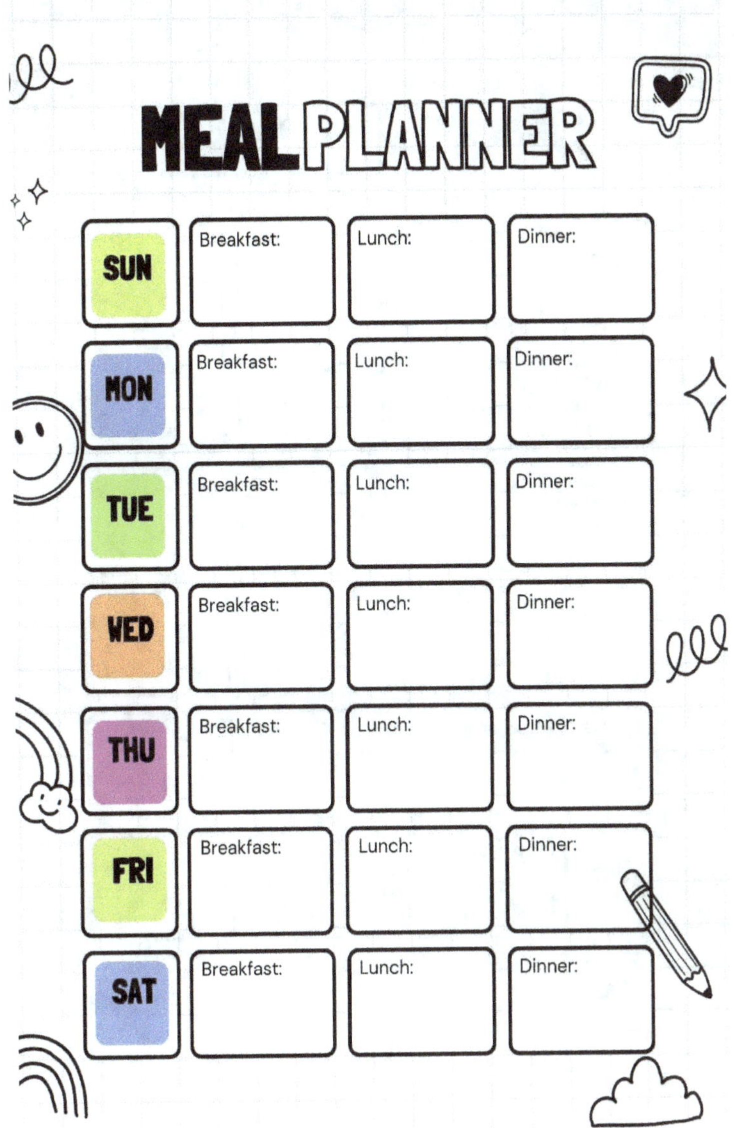

MEAL PLANNER
SUN
Breakfast:
Lunch:
Dinner:
MON
Breakfast:
Lunch:
Dinner:
TUE
Breakfast:
Lunch:
Dinner:
WED
Breakfast:
Lunch:
Dinner:
THU
Breakfast:
Lunch:
Dinner:
FRI
Breakfast:
Lunch:
Dinner:
SAT
Breakfast:
Lunch:
Dinner:

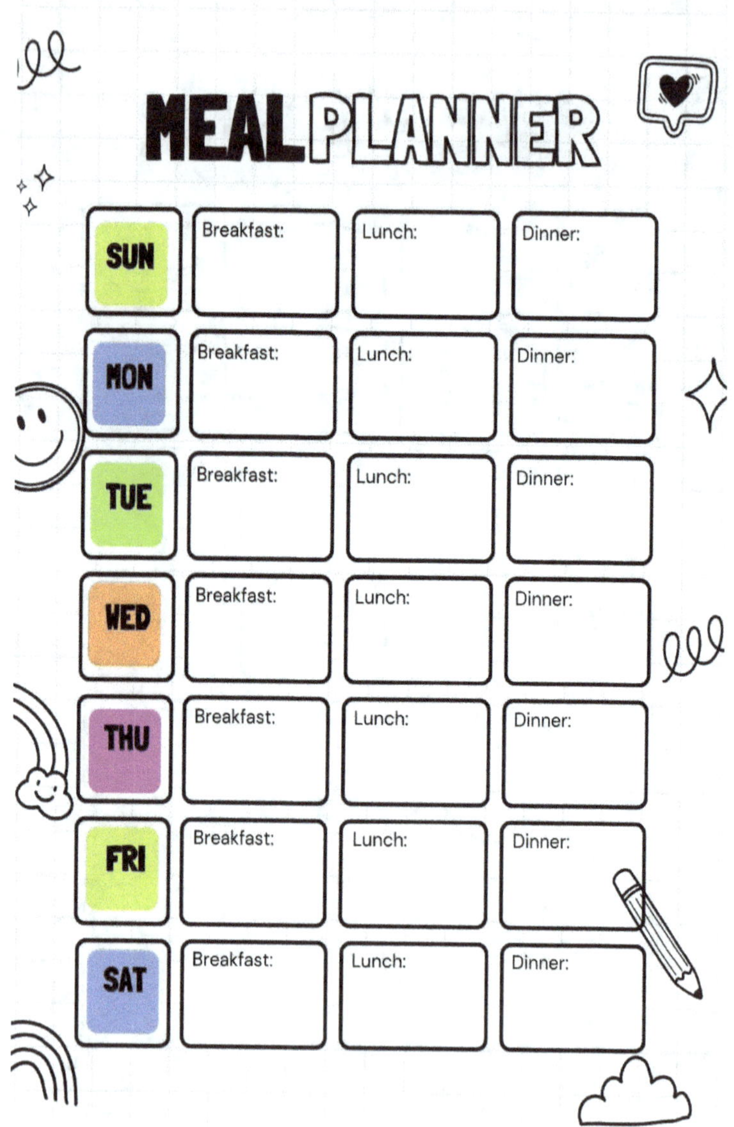
MEAL PLANNER
SUN
Breakfast:
Lunch:
Dinner:
MON
Breakfast:
Lunch:
Dinner:
TUE
Breakfast:
Lunch:
Dinner:
WED
Breakfast:
Lunch:
Dinner:
THU
Breakfast:
Lunch:
Dinner:
FRI
Breakfast:
Lunch:
Dinner:
SAT
Breakfast:
Lunch:
Dinner:

MEALPLANNER

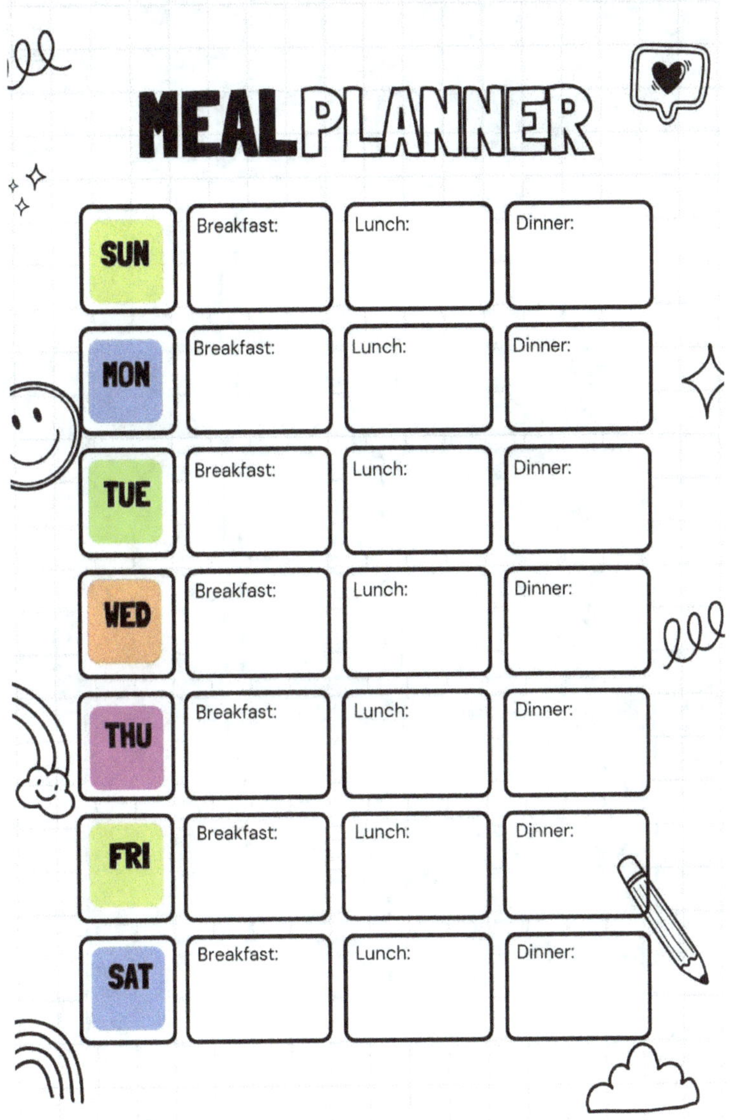

MEAL PLANNER

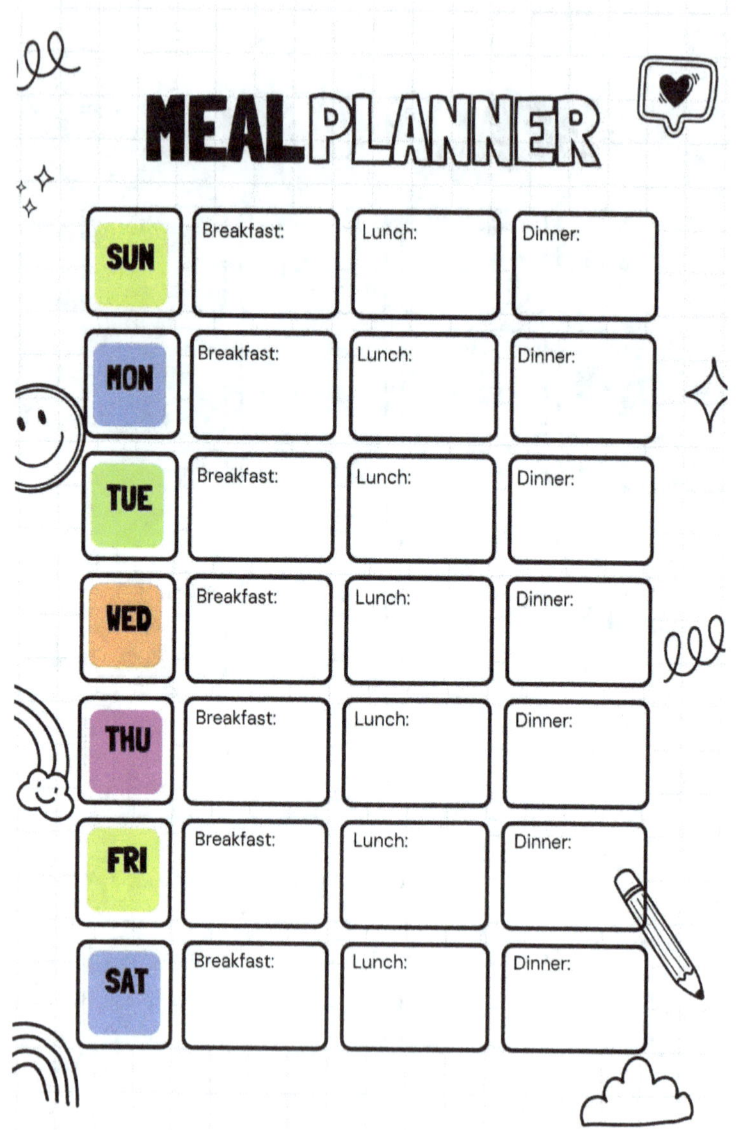